Natural Hair Revolution & Resolutions...

Kinky Hair Stories~ Continues

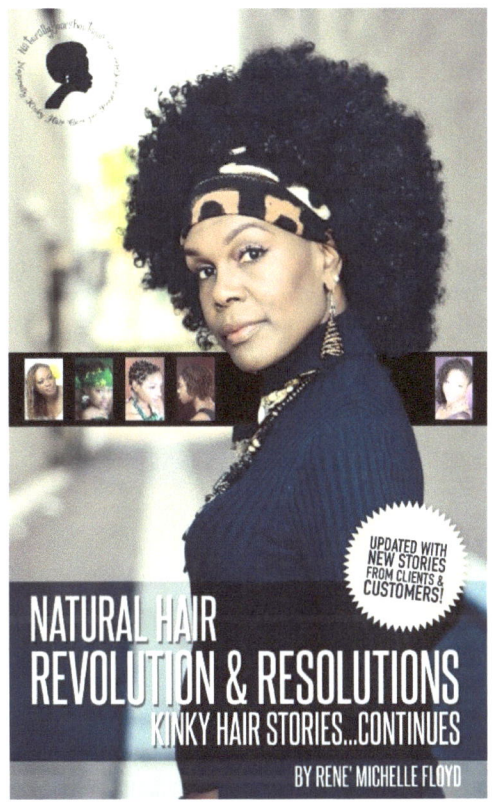

René Michelle Floyd

Dedication

I am dedicating this book to all the *natural heads* that took the leap and did the *BIG CHOP* and to those who are in the process of transitioning and who have already transitioned from wearing a perm to now wearing their own natural hair. Congratulations and welcome to the *natural hair world*.

A very special dedication goes out to my *little sister* who is a survivor of breast cancer; who lost her hair during chemotherapy treatments and now has a head full of beautiful natural hair—congratulations Chelsea D. Williams!

Disclaimer

The following stories are from my friends, family, clients and customers. The words and thoughts are their own, and in no way was solicited for gain of my business or the businesses of others.

In some of the text, if needed, the text was *slightly edited*, and in no way was intended to take away from the originality of the authors' stories.

==

WANT MORE?

For those of you who need more support and information about what it's like to 'go natural' and to learn more about natural hair care and tips and tricks, I cordially invite you to explore with us.

Submit your name and best email address to be included in our VIP Family for updates, private exclusive sales on Beautiful Hair Products and more!

SIMPLY CLICK THIS LINK BELOW

http://eepurl.com/cn3kOH

==

Acknowledgments

I'd like to thank every person that submitted their own unique and personal hair story. It is *your story* that has made this book possible.

I acknowledge and thank all those who encouraged me to come out with a *new and updated edition* of the original and popular book, **"Natural Hair Revolution & Resolutions...Kinky Hair Stories,"** it has been a hit among the natural hair community.

It was time to give others an opportunity to share their hair stories and hopefully encourage a *new community* of natural hair wearers-- that they are not alone in their pursuit to making a smooth transition from a chemical produced hair style to wearing their own natural hair and to simply *connect* and share with others who are enjoying their natural hair.

Foreword

Crystal James, MPA

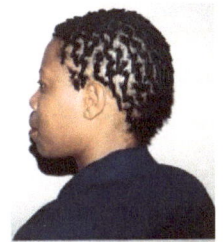
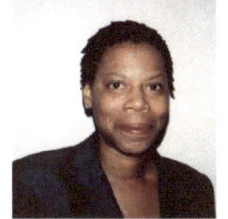

In 2005 I wrote about my experience with René Floyd at the very beginning of wearing and growing my natural hair. I still embrace my natural hair. I adore and respect my beautiful hair. The texture is extraordinary, unique, and very special. It is my own healthy, long and natural hair.

I respect my hair by not torturing it by straightening, weaving, or hiding it under wigs. I truly do not see how or why in 2014 that women subject their hair to hours of straightening for the appearance of "white" hair. I hated the restrictions my weaving, braiding, and straightening of my hair placed on my life.

The constant in my life is Rene' Floyd. She has been here from the beginning and in 2014 Rene' Floyd still sees the beauty of my natural hair. She has maintained my hair from the start and continues to do so in the present.

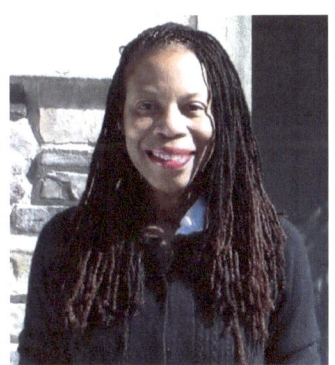
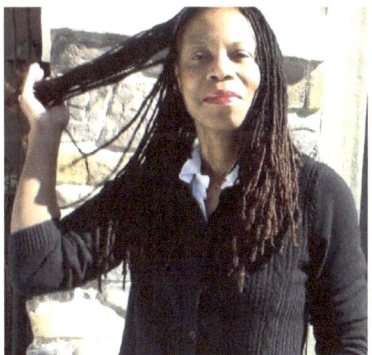
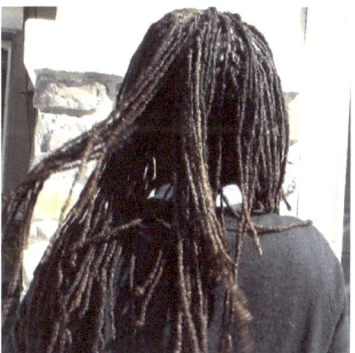

Her new book, **"Natural Hair Revolution & Resolutions...Kinky Hair Stories ~ Continues,"** is a small display of her talents and skills maintaining the beauty of natural hair. She has featured hair in calendars, several binders of beautiful photos of natural hair, a website, and I am sure many other displays. I love my hair and I owe that to Rene' Floyd.

Introduction

This edition of **Natural Hair Revolution & Resolutions...Kinky Hair Stories~ Continues** is an extension of the original book, **Natural Hair Revolution & Resolutions...Kinky Hair Stories**.

I've been in the (natural hair) business for a number of years now and after rendering services on hundreds of clients, I've come to the conclusion that my real business is that of sharing information with those individuals who are seeking ways to fall in love with their natural hair and learn how to take good care of it.

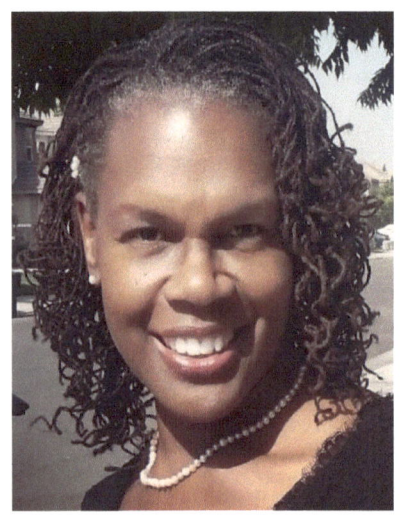 Essentially, I help others see the beauty in their own natural hair- no matter what you choose to call it; kinky, curly, coily or nappy—to me, it's all beautiful.

My job is to find out what your goal is for your hair— what's important to you and to help you arrive there. My main objective is to help you reach your goal in the most natural and healthiest way possible.

It doesn't matter what hair style you choose to wear; natural (unprocessed) hair, dreadlocks, Sisterlocks^{tm}, perm or buzz cut; whatever style you wear, whether or not you color your hair, whether you spend a grip on hair products or whether you're a DIY person, my number one mission is to help you have a more knowledgeable and informed journey...I am an *Information Philanthropist!*

So with that said, after 11 years, I thought it was time to render another book with NEW hair stories from new clients and friends that would both, inform and entertain you.

Following, you will find various stories from individuals who are either transitioning from a perm to wearing a natural hair style and telling why they did it or from those who've been natural for a long time and they simply want to share their natural hair journey and tell how they are enjoying it. The authors are excited about sharing why they love their natural hair style, and still others (who are my personal clients) freely express their appreciation for the services Naturally Yours Boutique has rendered to them over the years.

Many have come to the point of being free to be themselves and express how wonderful and liberating they feel.

The hair stories within these pages are stories of people just like you and me- people who have decided that enough is enough...they've taken their lives back and their money too. They've taken the time to share their stories with us. It is my hope that you enjoy and benefit from its content.

René Michelle Floyd, Author
Natural Hair Revolution & Resolutions...Kinky Hair Stories~ Continues
August 2014
Perris, California

Contents

What Is Hair?

Anatomy of a Hair

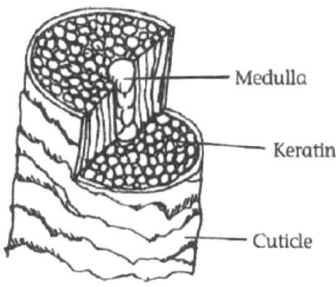

Medulla

Keratin

Cuticle

So, first of all, let's examine what hair is:

Hair is generally identified as a *class characteristic* not an individual characteristic.

Individual characteristic: can be related to a particular person or ethnicity.

Class characteristic: can be related to groups of people.

Hair grows from *hair follicles* located in the dermis—the skin; the thick layer of living tissue below the epidermis that forms the true skin of the scalp.

While hair is growing beneath the epidermis, its outer covering is soft. Once it goes past the epidermis, the outside layer hardens into keratin.

Inside the follicle, the hair is growing and is "connected" to blood vessels and nerves.

Outside the skin, the hair is essentially dead!

In the natural hair community, you will find some great information. People are now speaking out with authority on what *type of hair* they've been blessed with.

There are various ranges of curl patterns, from 1a – 4 c hair curl patterns.

For instance, if you fall into the category of having type 1a hair, your hair would be considered straight or fine/thin hair, while 1b type hair is considered medium/straight and has a little more body than 1a. On the other hand, if you fall into category number 2a, your hair is considered wavy fine/thin, while 2c is wavy/coarse.

There's still category 4, which ranges from 4a- kinky/soft, to 4b- kinky/wiry, to 4c- kinky/zingy.

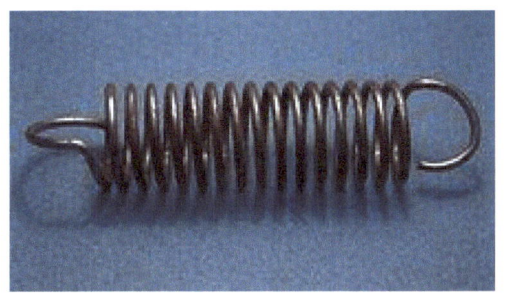 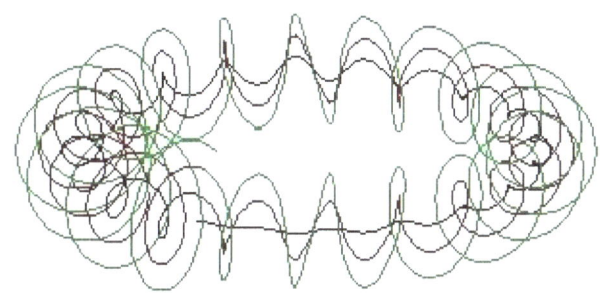

*Pictured images shows how the spiral of the '4' type textured hair looks

I can almost say without a doubt, most of the readers of this book, fall into the #4a – 4c category. I say that, only because, 4a – 4c hair type is the most challenging type of hair to manage and find a happy medium between hair care and hair styling options.

What "Good Hair" _Is Not!_

Before I go any further, let me say this. _Good hair_ is **NOT** isolated to any one particular race or group of people. **All <u>healthy hair</u> is _good hair_**. Each and every strand of your hair has its very own DNA. There are no two strands alike; and as various and diverse as human beings are, so is your hair—its texture, color and grade. So get excited about the fact that your hair in all its glory is your unique story!

The 'Good Hair' Movie—an observation

As a hair consultant and stylist, I was eager to watch the movie, "Good Hair", because I thought I was going to learn something new- something I didn't know before. Well, to say the least, I did!

I was appalled at the fact that Mr. Dudley knows that the chemical ingredients that make up for some of his hair products are very harmful to the health of the scalp, let alone the health of the individual who uses them. Yet, the Dudley Empire, owned and operated by black folks is estimated to be valued at around $35 million dollars, while the value of his Dudley product line is around $100 million dollars!

The _Dudley mansion_ and his manufacturing plant is located on forty-seven thousand beautiful acres and is valued at around $10 million—as it's said in the movie, " bad hair has been good business to the Dudley's.

I guarantee that Mr. Dudley doesn't care what I think or what you think for that matter. He is a business man and is capitalizing from the ignorance and oblivion of black folks—mostly black women.

The Black Hair Industry

The black hair industry is a *$9 BILLION dollar industry* and over 70% of the hair business is the *weave* hair business.

I can't speak too harshly because in years past, I fell into the rut of trying to look like my 'white' sisters; trying to achieve long hair by wearing long braids. I even wore long wigs at one time and went as far as getting a perm (that didn't take) and damaging my scalp, which caused major flaking of my scalp.

I know what it's like to read a label on a product jar in hopes that the *miracle* is on the inside and when it doesn't do what it espoused to do, buy the next *miracle jar*, still to no avail. And before I knew it, I'd have enough hair products in my cabinets to open up my own (used) beauty supply store!

In the movie, it pointed out that blacks buy triple the products than whites.

We spend a ton of money on products and hair; and for some, they skip paying their rent just to have 'good looking hair.'

There were a couple of stylists in the movie with beautiful dreadlocks; yet they were perming and weaving those clients and collecting that cash! To me, that's a double standard. The question is, are you in business to solely make money or are you in business to encourage our people to love their natural selves, starting with the hair on top of their heads?!

Now, I realize, that wearing your own natural hair—kinky, coily, wavy, nappy—whatever you want to call it—is not for everybody. It has been said, that wearing your own natural hair is a *calling.* I think the *calling* is from reevaluating what hair beauty really is.

I also realize that some people have medical issues they're dealing with that prevent them from wearing their own natural hair (if they have hair). Believe me; I know that a nice wig can save the day.

All I'm saying is, the hair industry is capitalizing from our insatiable consumption of hair and weaving products to the point of *killing* our own hair follicles (and never having a chance to wear our own hair again), to emptying our bank accounts in pursuit of looking like somebody else.

Mothers were getting their baby girls' hair permed at 3 and 4 and 5 years old!

The mentality of many young girls and women is that their hair is ugly and unless they have other people's hair in their heads, they don't feel beautiful— a very warped concept.

Our self-esteem is so low when it comes to our hair, that we're not realizing that the people that sell us the hair (Koreans and Chinese- maybe Japanese too) are laughing all the way to the bank.

It's time to wake up and look in the mirror and repeat the mantra, "I AM Beautiful just the way I am—hair and all." Clutch on to our money and save it for our bright future!

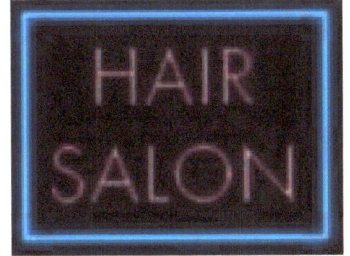

*The following poem is a classic from the original book. It was submitted by Barbara, my former client from Victorville, California—December 2003 I didn't want you to miss it, so I've included it in this edition…enjoy!

You Know It's A Black Salon When...

1. Your stylist accepts a 3-piece from Popeye's as her tip.

2. All the stylists walk around with house slippers on.

3. When your stylist takes a cigarette break; it's weed she smokes.

4. Your stylist is still there doing your hair even though she's supposed to be on bed rest.

5. Four people are booked for the same 1:00 appointment.

6. Your stylist calls YOU at the salon talkin' bout "I overslept, but I'm on my way."

7. When your stylist finally arrives—you can see that she had been to the club the night before because she still has on her club clothes, and she still has the red-- "over 21" stamp on the back of her hand.

8. Every hairstyle, no matter what you're getting, requires that nasty brown gel.

9. There's always that one stylist in the back that you can't tell whether it's a girl or a guy.

10. The STYLISTS' head looks a mess.

11. All the other stylists fake like someone else's clients hair looks good until they leave the shop and then it's—"Girl, I KNOW Shameeka ain't let her walk outta here like dat!"

12. There's a receptionist's booth at the front of the shop but no one ever uses it because it's stocked with beauty supplies.

13. The Asian man from the carryout across the street comes over and personally takes food orders.

14. Some crack head is always coming into the shop every five minutes trying to sell some deodorant or batteries.

15. You have to divide your tips 'bout four different ways cuz' one permed you, one shampooed you, one wrapped you and your stylist finished you up.

16. You get to the salon and your stylist isn't there, so you gotta page her. When she calls back, you gotta go pick her and her baby up.

17. Your ears are ringing because 'loud music' is playing on your stylists' radio and she is singing along.

18. Somebody is making a chicken run and is taking orders-- from the stylists AND the clients.

19. They got strawberry, orange, AND grape soda in the coke machine, but no coke.

20. Your stylist stops doing your hair to go outside and talk to her baby daddy.

21. Your stylist got 10 Polaroid pictures from the club stuck around the mirror.

22. Your stylist holds a 15-minute phone conversation with somebody while she styles your hair.

23. The tape man is there selling bootleg tapes for $5.

24. The owner of the shop and one of the stylists get into a cussing match in front of the customers cause she made an appointment after 5, knowing that she has to perform later that night.

25. The stylists all talk about each other.

26. When they send Boo-Boo's baby girl to the 99-cent store to buy your $10 "deep conditioner".

27. When the stylist's boyfriend comes in the shop with his boys and you are just hoping that they hurry up with your hair before it's a drive-by.

28. When, for a finishing touch, your stylist insists on sprinkling a little bit of glitter in your hair.

29. When your entire day is on hold because you have a hair appointment. Appointment is for 9:00a.m. Your stylist arrives at 10:30 a.m. -- She gets to you around 11:30 a.m. --Goes to lunch at 12:00 noon—Comes back around 2:00p.m. and eats lunch while doing your hair. --Sends Lil' Ray Ray to the store for some conditioner at 3:30p.m. —Puts you under the dryer at

4:00p.m.—Takes you from under the dryer at 5:00p.m.—Starts styling your hair at 6:00p.m. and finishes up around 8:00 p.m.

Chelsea D. Williams

My name is Chelsea and I am the queen of versatility when it comes to hairstyles! I have had long hair, short hair, colored hair, permed hair, shaved hair, kinky hair and no hair at all! The photos that you see are some of my hair metamorphosis.

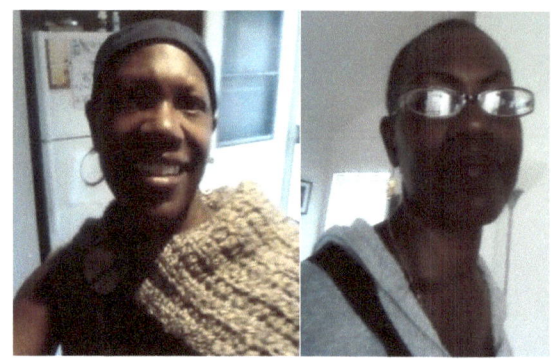

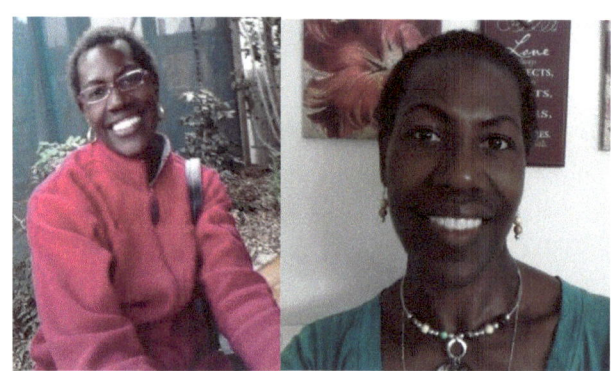

In 2011 I was diagnosed with breast cancer and I underwent several treatments of chemotherapy. After the second treatment of chemo, my hair began to fall out. I asked my husband to shave it for me. Cutting my hair was my attempt to taking control of the hair loss, and not allowing the hair loss take control of me. So, I was sporting scarfs, wigs and cute skull caps for about 7 months before my hair began to grow back. Boy was I excited! I swore to myself that I would only wear my hair natural and would not burden my scalp or my system with harmful chemicals from perms or hair dyes again.

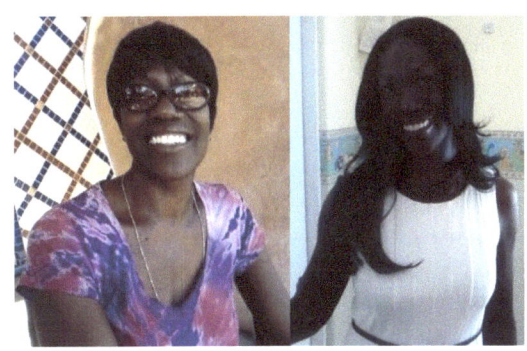

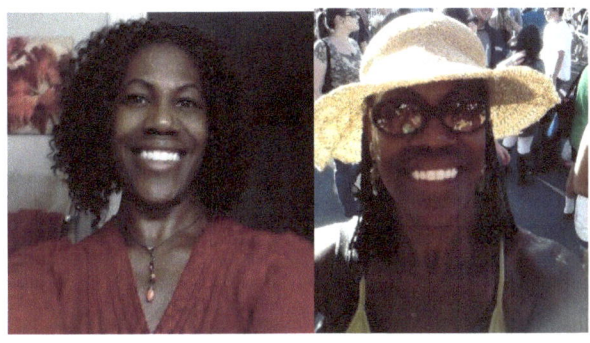

As my hair began to grow back, I was not ready to embrace the grey stands that sprinkled my mane. I committed myself to researching natural hair color alternatives. The best option that I found was henna.

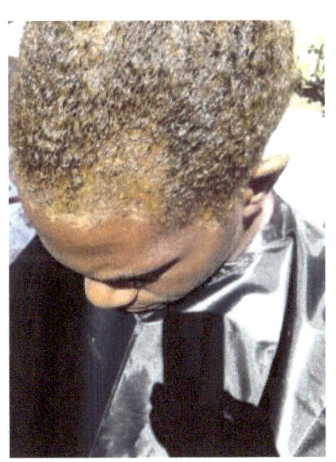
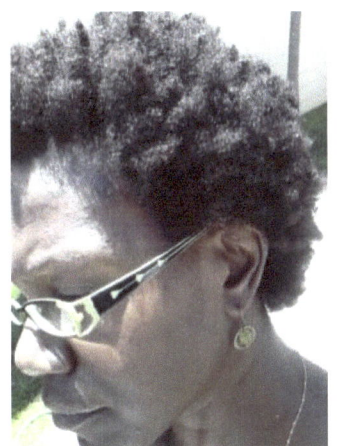
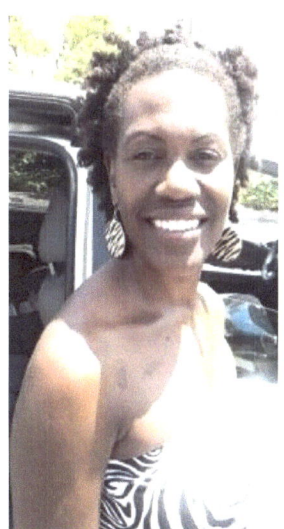

Henna is a 100% plant based hair color that works great for me. As you can see, I am in love with my natural, kinky hair and its texture.

I am so happy to be natural! I feel liberated and free!

Tyra Robinson of Indigenous Curls

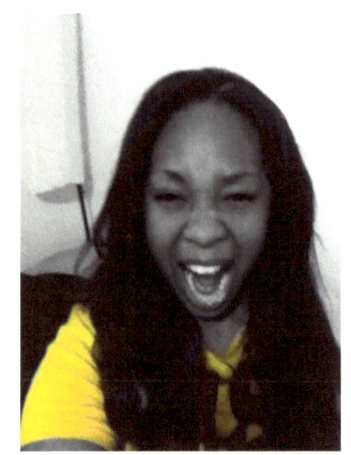

When I Big Chopped, I was a few months into a new relationship. For years I rocked waist long weaves, huge fluffy wigs, or braids, while my own hair was crying out for attention. I spent months researching, and planning how I would transition, what styles I would rock, and how to maintain the new style. I was ready to make a change, but scared of the possible results.   One day, I came home, frustrated with life. I sat on the edge of my bed, & took out my weave. "I need a change," I kept telling myself, as I unraveled each braid. 30mins later the weave was gone, but I was unsatisfied.

 My hair was a dry, dull mess. I took a long look in the mirror, examining every strand. I loved how my 2 inches of new growth had so much life, Kink, & shine. But the rest of the hair strand looked limp & lifeless. Without another thought chopped off all my relaxed ends, and hopped in the shower. There I stood, with nothing to hide behind, no weave, and no makeup, just me. Minutes later my boyfriend came over…….

"Oh Shit" He howled, as his eyes connected with my new do.

"You like it?!" I asked excitedly.

"What you 'bout to do with IT?" he asked, His face had "concern" written all over it.

"Nothing…" My heart sank. Not the answer I was looking for….

"I can rock some big beautiful earrings, and headbands---"he cut me off

"No Weave?" he asked, as he took a seat, breathing deeply.

"I have to get used to IT" He said, as his eyes bounced around my hair.

My feelings were hurt. He could of lied, and left my feelings intact. Hindsight is 20/20. Today I appreciate his honesty.

We had a group outing planned the following weekend, but he canceled, sighting fatigue. I had a feeling it was my new do. As weeks, passed, I noticed a change in our dynamic. Once extremely affectionate, he began to become distant. He used to walk with his arm around me, post BC, he would barley hold my hand in public. I began to feel as if my hair wasn't good enough. I noticed his eyes would travel to girls who still rocked their long weaves. Occasionally he would point out hairstyles on other girls he liked. They were all flat glossy weaves. 2 months after BC I began to develop a complex, between his side comments, and the surprising reaction from my Mother. I felt insecure, and started regretting my decision. I purchased a (hideous) full lace wig, and hid under that for 2 weeks. My Boyfriends response:

"You look like 'You' again!" He was excited, and immediately offered to go out on a date. I smiled and agreed, but I was boiling inside.

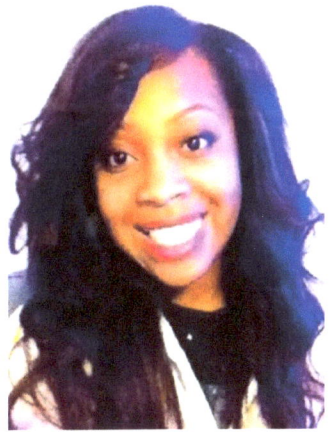

Did he only like me for my unauthentic appearance? Why was he only affectionate & romantic when I had an 18 inch weave? His true roots were starting to show & I didn't like it one bit. Needless to say, we broke up, and I was happily single!

Time passed, and I was sitting on the edge on my bed, once again, in dire need of a change. I had been rocking braids 6 months post BC. I had also started dating someone new. His hair was locked, and he fully understood the needs of natural hair. He seen the beauty of my coils and complimented even the most shrunken wash & goes. His family introduced me to natural hair products.

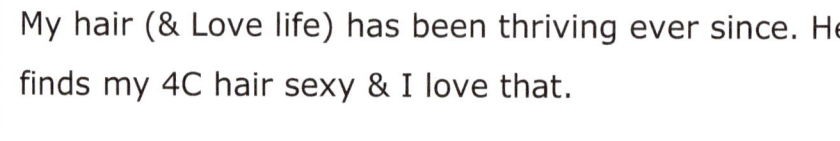

My hair (& Love life) has been thriving ever since. He finds my 4C hair sexy & I love that.

My experience with dating & big chopping, may or may not be unique. What was your experience? Was it well received? Do you attract a different type of person depending on your style? Ladies Weigh in!

Traci Baty

Since before my teens, I have always wished for long, silky, beautiful hair. I was about 10 or 11 years old when I got my first perm. I remember looking at the lady on the box and thinking my hair would be just as Beautiful. No Such Luck!

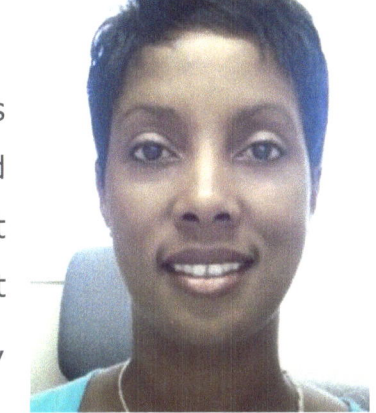

When I was younger, I would sometimes go 6 months or more in between perms and my hair suffered tremendously. My mom, not knowing at the time that proper maintenance was important to prevent breakage, just labeled me as having her hair texture, 'BAD'!

For as long as I can remember, the hair above my ears would grow just below my earlobes while the rest was much shorter and noticeably uneven. The breaking and shedding became a never-ending cycle.

During the summer months, in the stifling Texas heat, I would wear a head scarf around my hair so I didn't have to look at or deal with it. I often felt like Cinderella before the ball. Lol!

I took cosmetology for two years in high school and after graduation I enrolled in Vogue Beauty School. I felt this would give me a better understanding on how to properly care for my hair. As one can imagine, there wasn't anything we didn't try at least once.

When Jody Watley hit the scene I was totally infatuated with her hair. I had to have her look by any means possible so this was my introduction to 'The Weave'. Remember her video 'Looking for a New Love'? That video was the inspiration for my new hairstyle. One of the top students at Vogue did my hair and I was thrilled and horrified at the same time. The thrill came from seeing myself for the first time with wavy "good" hair that draped my shoulders. The horror came from the fact that I had so much additional hair on my head I could barely hold it up. I do believe the creator of the 'Bobble Head' dolls saw me walking around one day and to their amusement came up with a clever idea. LOL!

Over the years the perms and weaves continued to thin out and damage my hair. At one salon visit I told the stylist that I was concerned about possible over processing in the crown section of my head. I told her it felt like I had a little breakage. She seemed a little embarrassed when she told me that in fact it looked like I was actually going bald. I heard myself shouting, 'BALD as in like a Man, BALD?' She politely whispered, 'Yes.' LAWDT, Please don't let this happen, I was too young to go bald. I didn't want to walk around wearing wigs for the rest of my life.

After that visit, I started massaging my scalp and I would perm the top of my head last so I wouldn't have to leave it on too long. The hair in that area slowly started growing back but it was still rather thin. For the majority of my adult life I wore my hair cut in a short Halle Berry style, if I allowed it to grow longer it ended up stringy and uneven. I kept the top a little longer because I literally had to do a comb over to cover the thin area in my crown. I wore a Donald Trump before Donald Trump.

Three times the charm. After the third try, I can finally say, I will NEVER go back to the creamy crack. The first time I went back to the perm because of peer pressure. I heard it all from, 'You're not pretty enough to wear that style' to, 'Are you going through an emotional period in life?'

The second time was because of lack of knowledge. I didn't know anything about my natural hair, I was clueless. I live in a town that's not really considered small but there weren't any natural stylists. Before I did my third and Final Big Chop, I did TONS of research on Natural Hair. I read articles, blogs, website's and watched YouTube videos. Most of all, I was determined to be the person God created and to love ALL of me including my hair.

My last perm was on October 13, 2010 and I have never been happier with my hair. I've always thought my hair was ugly, thin and lifeless when in reality it wasn't my hair. It was the damaging effects of the perm. My crown is still thin but it is barely noticeable.

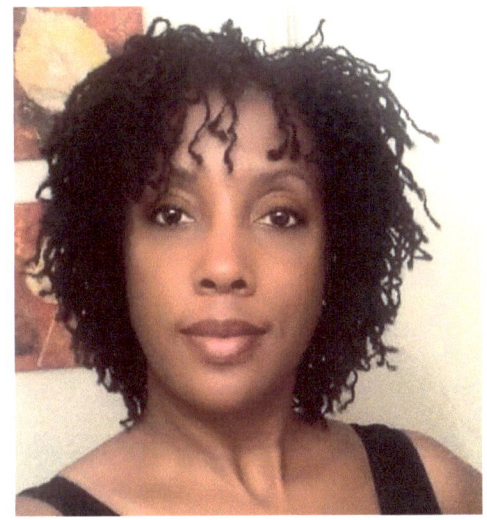

On February 14, 2012, after another intensive research, I got Sisterlocks™ as a Valentine gift to myself. My initial research was on Interlocks and somehow I ran across Sisterlocks™. All I can say is, God makes no mistakes. I've had my SL's for 26 months and I am Finally IN LOVE with my hair. Who would have thought the little girl who once prayed that her hair turned out exactly like the lady's hair on the perm box would ever love the hair she once dreaded.

Yes, I do have gray hair but at this time I have chosen not to accept it. Maybe in another decade. Lol!

Wilhelm Davidson

After many years of wearing my hair in a short or fade hairstyle and going to the barbershop on a weekly or bi-weekly schedule, I decided I wanted to try a different or low maintenance hairstyle. I always said I would never wear a dreadlock or loc hairstyle because of the negative connotations or stereotypes that society associated with this hairstyle.

At one time in my life, I thought anyone wearing Locs was not into healthy grooming or proper hair maintenance. I often wondered how anyone could wash and keep this style of hair clean.

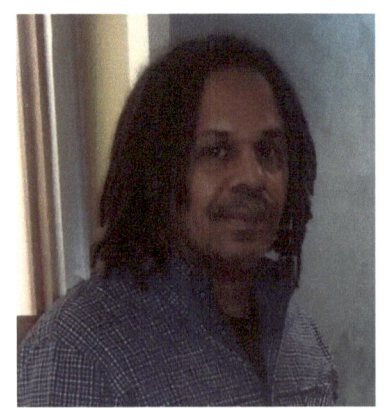 As I entered middle age and feeling less concerned of what society thought, I said to myself why not give this loc hairstyle a try and if I did not like it I had the option of cutting it and going back to my previous hairstyle. So, In January 2011, I decided I wanted to go with Locs but first I needed to grow-out my hair. I began getting my hair braided at a local hair braiding shop so it would have the proper length to begin twisting.

I first started wearing my hair in a twisted style for a few months before I was ready to begin my hair loc journey. Every 4 to 6 weeks, my loctician would re-twist my hair. There are many ways I can wear my hair with Locs so I change it up from time to time with braids or half twist styles.

I had done numerous researches and watched countless YouTube videos, so I could be as well informed or educated as possible on how to properly maintain and care for them. My Locs have also helped me to feel more self-confident and less concerned with what others thought.

I truly love my Locs and anyone who wears Locs will admit that they take on a personality of their own. There are days when they may look great and other days when they are frizzy or not looking so great but I just take it all in stride. I doubt that I would have worn Locs earlier in my career with the workforce being less accepting of them but now many professionals such as doctors, teachers and even policeman wear them.

Locs are still looked down upon by many people but I have learned not to be concerned with conservative or narrow minded thinking people. I've been wearing Locs for 3 years and I am so glad I made this choice to wear them. This is my natural hair story.

Asabi Nzingha Alexander

My mother had a rough hair journey. When she had children of her own she felt that having healthy hair was very important. Because she had so many

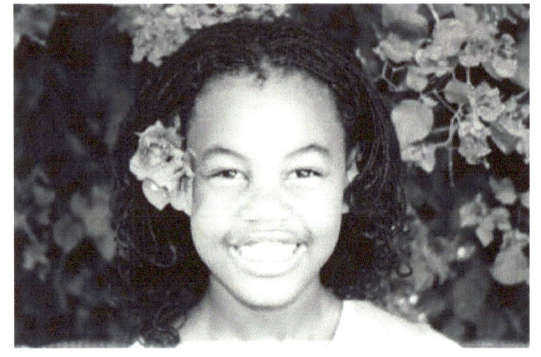

kids, doing our hair everyday wasn't something she had time for, so she gave us all dread locks. Somewhere down the road she cut all of our locks out and we started over with loose natural hair.

Then her attention was set on this new hair style called, Sisterlocks^{tm}. She fell in love with them and so did I. I was

the one to really encourage her to learn how to do the hair style because I wanted them. I was only 5 years old at the time when I asked her to learn.

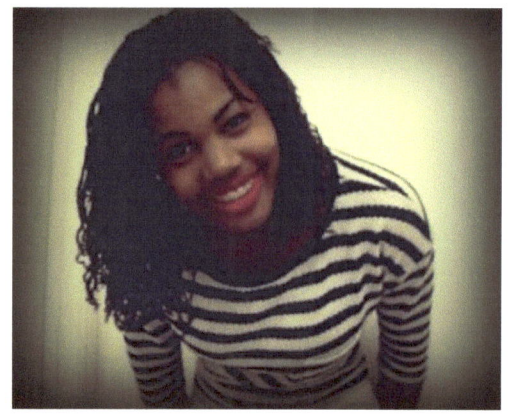

Soon after she learned how to do the particular style of Sisterlocks^{tm}, I was her

first client. Since the age of 5 I grew my locks out until the age of 18. Then I big chopped on March 26, 2014. The reason behind me doing the big chop is

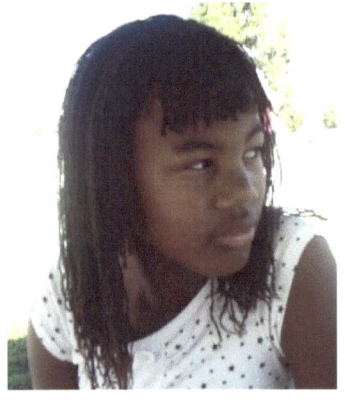

because my locks were all uneven and they were not growing how I wanted them to.

During the summer of 6th grade I decided that I wanted to cut myself some bangs. At the time I really enjoyed having bangs but in the long run having bangs hindered me. As time went by my hair became more and more uneven. I decided to try and even out my hair by cutting portions around my head. That was the biggest mistake I could have ever made. Ever since I cut my hair those two times, my hair seemed to never grow back.

From middle school all the way until my senior year in high school my hair stayed the same length.

My two sisters also had Sisterlocks[tm] as well and they cut theirs off before I cut mine. When they cut their hair off it influenced me to believe that I could do it to.

September 16th was when I started to transition from Locs to loose natural hair. During my transition stage I frequently braided my hair to try and blend the roots with the Locs. It blended well for the first half of my 6 month transition. The second half of my transition was a challenge because there was so much new growth and it was harder to blend.

On March 26, 2014 at 2:30 pm is when I officially big chopped. I can honestly say I have no regrets in big chopping because now I can be versatile in the hair styles I wear.

Ollie Eubany

I love my Sisterlocks^{tm}—I am always ready to go out; no fuss, no mess, and they always look good.

I remember back in high school when I had to take a swimming course, I had an understanding teacher who took us black girls aside and told us she understood why we were reluctant to get into the pool. She knew we had straightened our hair. She told us to buy a Shammy, which would go under out bathing cap—it helped only a little as my hair did *go back*.

Then came the perm – I did my first perm myself with a perm I purchased

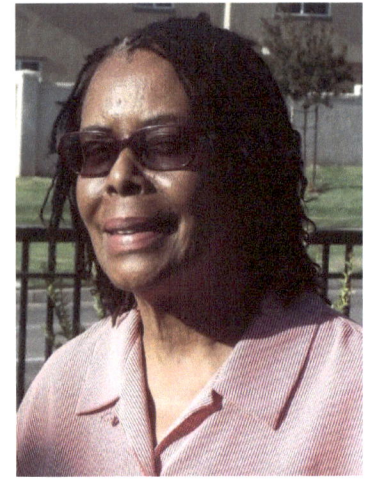

from the supermarket. I just did not put on the activator—result, I lost all my hair. I wore wigs for years. Then came the Jerri-curl, which was great for a while, but I noticed my hair was thinning—back to my wigs.

At church one day in October 2006 while talking to the usher he said he was writing a book on black hair and he had interviewed a lady who did Sisterlocks^{tm}. I got the telephone number and even without any research I made an appointment and it was the best decision I could make. Now my locks have grown and I have a really special loctician, René Michelle Floyd.

I so enjoy my locking sessions with her every 8 weeks and when she finishes locking she applies a spray on my hair, rubs it through and I can feel my locks glowing.

Sikudhani Alexander

My name is Sikudhani Alexander and here is my natural hair story. I've been blessed with being natural all my life. I never desired a perm and I still don't. My mother used to always do our hair the way we wanted whether long braids, short twists or an Afro.

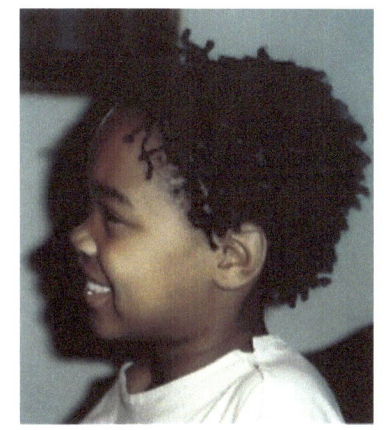

Going to a predominantly white school my hair was always a topic for discussion. One day my mother caught wind of a permanent natural hairstyle called Sisterlocks^{tm} and she never looked back. Both of my sisters were dying to have them in their head, but I was the only one who didn't care for them. At that time I didn't have a choice of what I would do with my hair. Soon after my mother decided to put them in my hair.

Growing up I found them awkward to style and hard to like. With the heartless middle school kids teasing relentlessly and making fun of my hair calling me

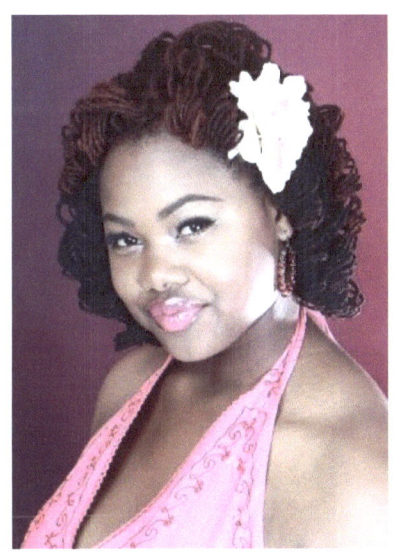

Bob Marley and other loc wearers wasn't helping either. I just didn't want them in my hair but I wasn't old enough to take them out by choice. The age of choice was 16. The funny thing is after I turned 16 I didn't take them out and I began embracing them.

They were so thick long and beautiful by the time I was 19. One day my older sister showed up to church shocking everyone with her new short permed Halle Berry cut. I couldn't stop staring at her hair and at that moment I knew it was time to make a change. I didn't know how or when but I knew it had to happen soon. When my birthday rolled around she told me she wanted to do something special and she knew how much I wanted to cut my hair so she said she would pay for a cut, perm and style. I was over the moon excited and I agreed. Then I realized I don't want a perm but I still want it cut. Not too short of course because at this time I was used to longer hair. So I decided to just pick out my locks so that I could save some length.

Seven whole days and two swollen thumbs later, my hair was loose. I was so excited but then I didn't know what to do. I didn't research like I should've and I felt crippled and ugly.

So I started covering up my hair with braids weaves and even wigs. Then I tried again to style my natural hair and it was just limp with so many split ends and damage. I hated it.

One day I decided that at some point I'm cutting all my hair off but I didn't know when. So I got braids with a shaved side. I loved those but I decided that after those I'm cutting my hair. I was waiting to get money to go to a barber shop and get it cut. Then I realized how dumb that was and how much time I was wasting. That weekend I was going to visit my parents. So that Thursday morning I woke up, got scissors and chopped all of my hair off. Then I got the trimmer forgetting that I'm not a barber and went to shave slightly and nicked my head. At that point I was taken aback and realized I had to literally be bald. I took a deep breath and began shaving until all of my hair was on the sink. I was in a rush so I tied some random weave tracks to the bottom of my head with a scarf and darted out the door.

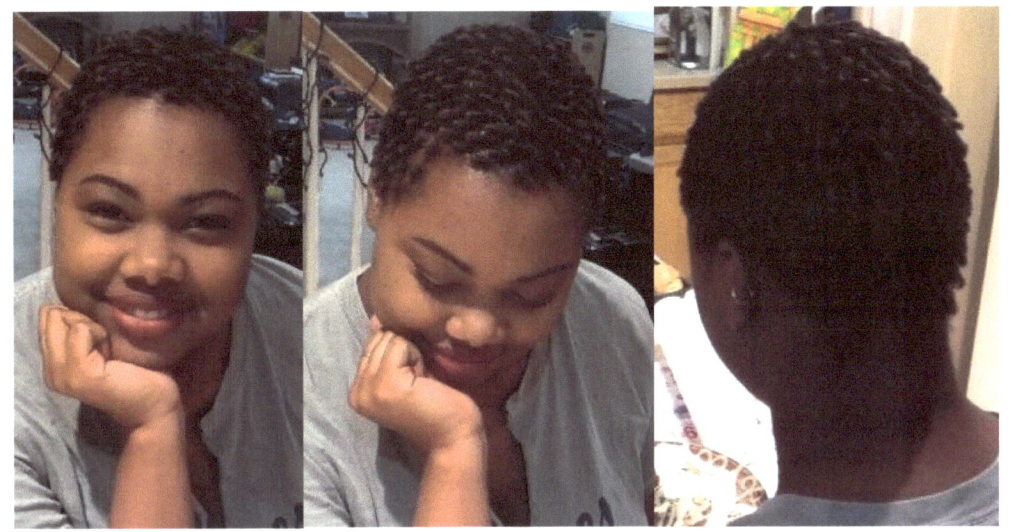

When I got to my parents' house I told my mom, grandma and sister to come with me and then pulled my scarf off and revealed my bald head. The first thing my mom said was "you have a nice head" Lol. Then my little sister's mouth dropped open and my grandma admired it. At that point I felt better but I wasn't ready to go out with my head like that yet. So my little sister made a custom wig for me out of Malaysian hair and it came out beautifully but since the base for the wig was a shower cap it made my head sweat and uncomfortable but it was either wear that wig or wear my scalp so I grinned and bearded it.

After only a couple weeks the wig was falling apart and I knew I had to do something, so my uncle bought me a lace front wig. It was a nice short human hair wig with little to no volume Lol but I rocked it. I started embracing my short haircut but I had just started school and since I showed up the first day with a wig I have to finish out the semester with it. My hair started growing, I developed a regimen and 4 months later I was wigless.

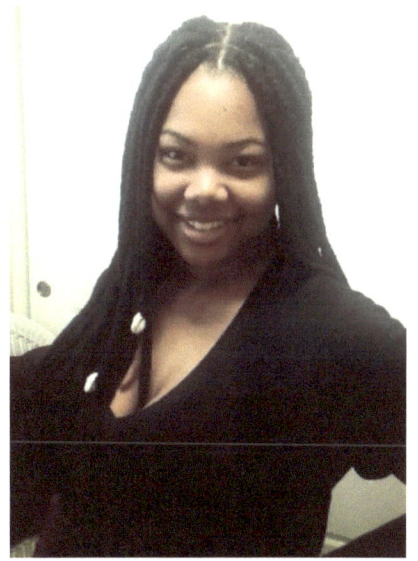

After that I decided to color it and I rocked that for about six months. A couple of weeks ago I decided to go back to black and I currently have a protective style--yarn braids, in my hair that my mother did and I love it!

I will be celebrating my 8 month post big chop anniversary on the 8th of April and it's only up from here. I am loving my loose natural hair and my journey is beautiful! I literally learn something new every day.

I am looking forward to getting back to my hair being down my back again; but I am enjoying the ride and the road that it takes to get there! Thank you so much for reading my journey!

Phyllis Brown

I am proud to be an African American woman. I recall when I was young, wanting and wishing to be 'white' or have long flowing hair. I grew up in the era where only a few black people, if any, were on T.V. we also played with blond hair, blue-eyed dolls.

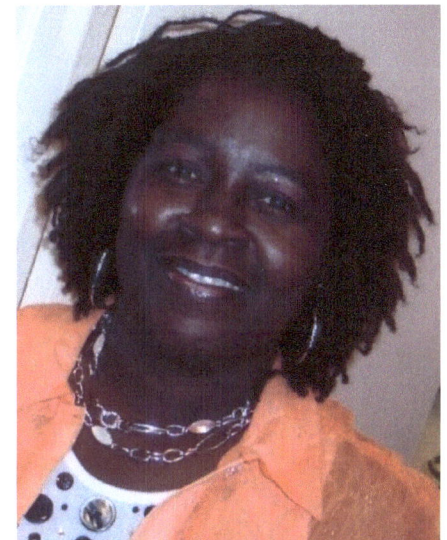

As I became a teenager I was proud of my natural hair. When afros first came out, I used lotion to curl my hair and make a curly afro for our first black history day.

My mom was against afros at the time, and washed and pressed my hair out when I got home from school. At least I got to wear it for the first black history day. Didn't see an afro until say it loud made us proud; thanks James Brown ☺

I wore perms and that always broke my hair off eventually, and I got tired of having a burnt scalp. My hair is thick and beautiful and always wore well in any style.

I started wearing different braided hairstyles for a while. One day I saw a young lady with a beautiful head of hair. It looked like a curly afro style from afar. As she got closer to me, I noticed they were little braids, which turned out to be called Sisterlocks[tm].

I thought, well I always wear braids, so this must be a good style for me. I experimented with the 2 braid twists with my own hair for a while to make sure that was the permanent style I wanted. I always received good compliments about my hair.

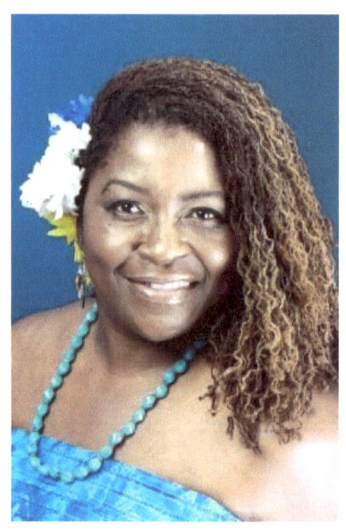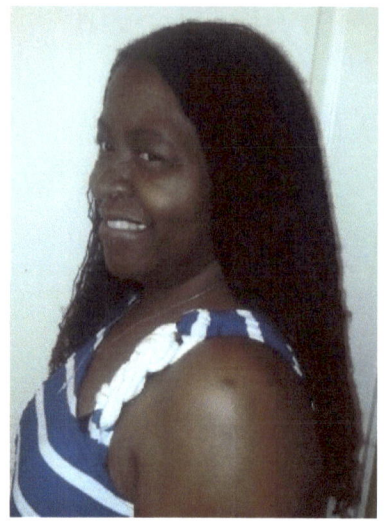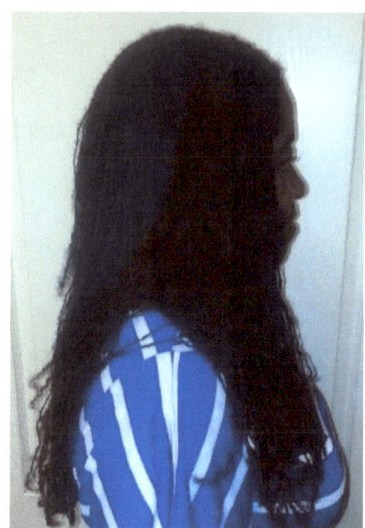

Then I was introduced to René, my consultant. She had a Sisterlocks party with JoAnn Cornwell as guest. She had beautiful long locks. So many different styles and lengths and colors; gorgeous, were they also. I had to wait another month for a consultation. I was so anxious, could hardly wait. Then my journey began 8 ½ years ago. It took two long days to install, but worth the wait. So happy; this was the best hair decision I could have made. Proud to be a natural Sisterlocks^{tm} woman. We stand alone in the natural hair arena, which makes us very special and unique. I love, love, love, my long natural hair.

I always think back to when I was a child and wanted to be white and have long hair. God gave me everything I needed from the beginning. I have no need to be white, because black is who I am, and hair was always there. Now it's long also. What a blessing to be me and Sister locked.

Thanks René!

Reneka Gibbs

I began wearing Sisterlocks^{tm} in August 2006, a few months after my first child was born. I was a new mom and wanted as much free time as possible

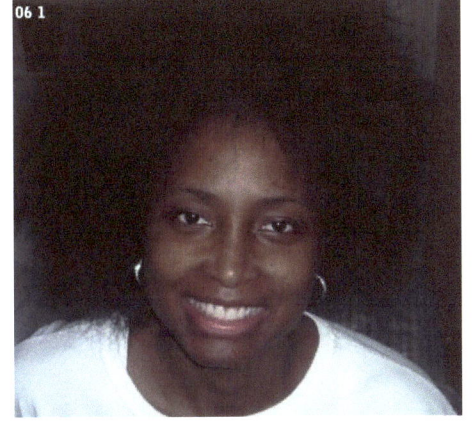

in order to begin my journey of motherhood.

Before Sisterlocks^{tm} I wore relaxers, press-ncurls and braids. Between my hair breaking off after a relaxer, spending countless hours and dollars in a hair salon, and struggling to find someone to braid my hair, I had had enough.

After having kids I couldn't imagine keeping up with this lifestyle. I had researched Sisterlocks^{tm} for a long time before this and felt it was time for me to adjust to my locks. I do not regret my decision to go all natural.

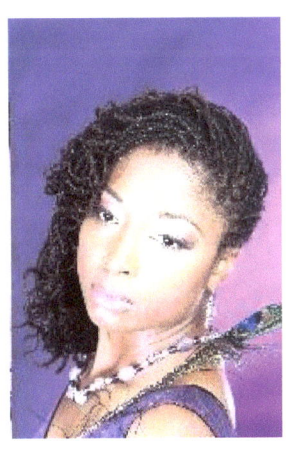 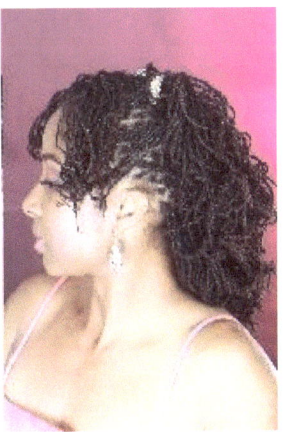 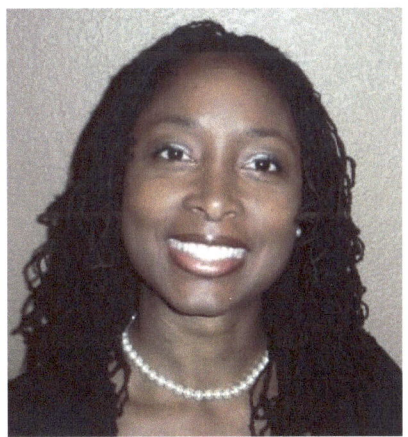

I now have the freedom to sweat, swim and shower without worrying about my hair.

Sisterlocks^{tm} has given me a new found confidence in my hair with an ease and versatility that I hope to embrace for a lifetime.

Jessie Smith

I am/was a barber. I learned to cut my hair and my brother's hair as early as elementary. I used to cut my hair as many as 3 times a week to "keep it tight."

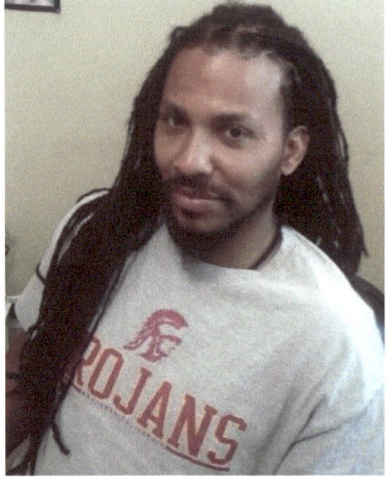

One day in '99 (in which I hadn't cut my hair in about 2 weeks), I got the idea I would let my hair grow. Not knowing for how long or even in what direction. Certainly Locs weren't even on my mind back then as I was about 19 years old.

Eventually I started to have my hair braided as I was still 'trying to figure out' what to do with my hair. At this time braids became a fad and everywhere I looked everyone had braids and I knew it was time to figure it out or cut it off.

Suddenly, like a ray of sunshine, I started noticing this style for which I had always assumed previously was only associated with being Jamaican and having to smoke weed to pull off.

This style is of course, Locs. I fell in love with it and I knew it was gonna be my look in the near future.

I started by having my already lengthy hair twisted. This didn't last long as I learned I couldn't wash my hair as often as I chose. And that could be a terrible result as I was very active and my scalp was constantly sweating under the summer sun; plus the smell...yeah. We'll leave that one alone.

After 6 months of this 'start up' I ran into someone that introduced me to 'brother Locs.' I was skeptical at first, but it was the best decision I could do for my Locs. This was 2003 after over 3 years of braids. Now, almost 15 years of hair growth, I have lots of Locs.

April Morgan

My name is April and I am proud of my five year journey wearing Sisterlocks^{tm}.

When women go through a self-awareness change such as I did in 2009, the first change I wanted was drastic. I wanted to shed the artificial layers and decided to take out the 20 inch weave, cut all the perm out, and begin with virgin hair.

I had did my research through the Sisterlocks^{tm} website for my husband's Brotherlocks installation 3 years prior and really loved his transformation, but 22 hours after my installation I could not believe I actually said good-bye to the 'creamy crack', and the Yaki weave, and honestly, it took me 3 years to thoroughly appreciate my freedom.

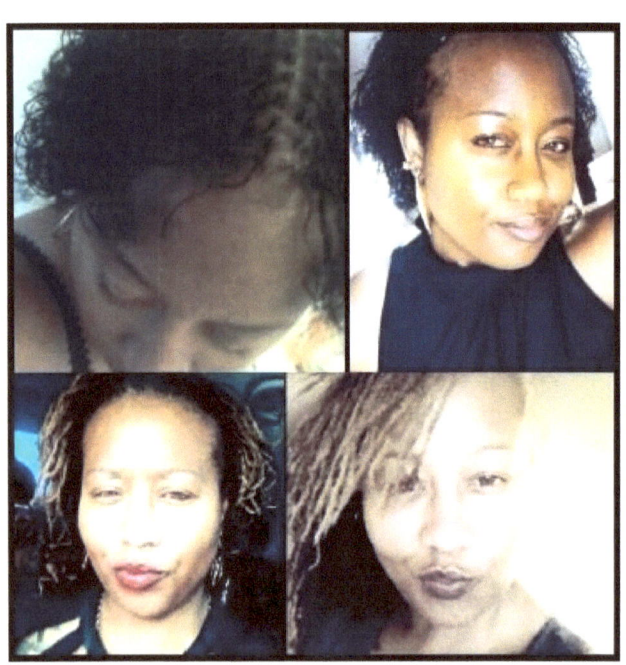

The transition was a permanent decision, made in a temporary circumstance,
and 5 years later, I will never look back.

When miss René initially did my install, my Locs were identifiable because she finesses each lock with her tools, and they lay so luscious and natural.

People who are in the Sisterlocks^{tm} community can distinguish Locs by Naturally Yours Boutique

40

automatically.

Due to my schedule, I opted to utilize the service of another Certified Sisterlocks^{tm} consultant, but my journey was made possible by the hands of René Floyd, who I am grateful to be a part of her sisterhood.

Kerry Morgan

My name is Kerry and I proudly wear my Brotherlocks going on 8 years in

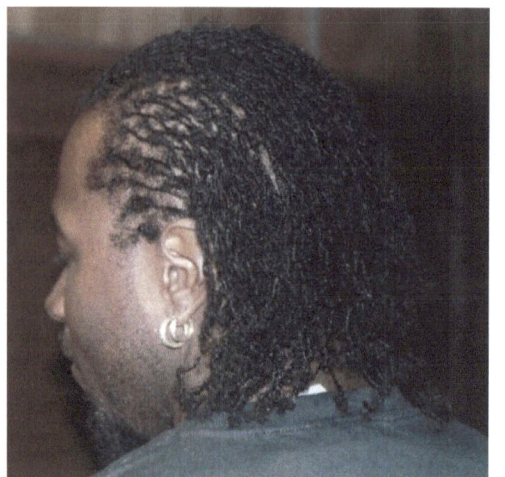

December. Transitioning into Brotherlocks was the best decision I have ever made. I had worn long hair primarily all my life and was over, looking for braiders, or braiders that didn't rip my hair out, or braiders who gave me styles with beads that didn't fit my age, or style.

When I initially started Locs, I was unhappy with the style of Locs and began reading up on the locking process and was thoroughly disappointed with the 'mess' in my head, which was nothing like the Brotherlocks I saw on the Sisterlocks™ website.

My Brotherlocks installation was the foundation of my growth. I found that you must research and choose a Certified Sisterlocks™ consultant in order to achieve proper and tremendous growth of your Brotherlocks, otherwise you just have 'whodunit' Locs.

Since Naturally Yours Boutique installed my Locs, the education began at my test Locs appointment and every

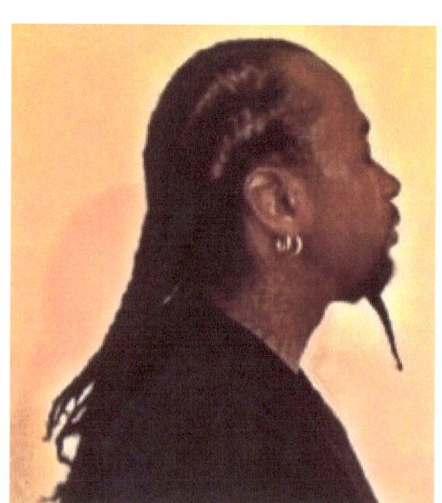

appointment thereafter. Mrs. Floyd, gives tips on maintenance, natural chemical-free products to use, and even gives me a fresh braided style to enhance my long Brotherlocks.

I can't see wearing my hair in any other way.

Wanda Irby

I recently had turned 50 years old and graduated to become an RN. I have worn pressed hair, permed hair, weaved hair and braids for many years. My hair and hairline were severely damaged.

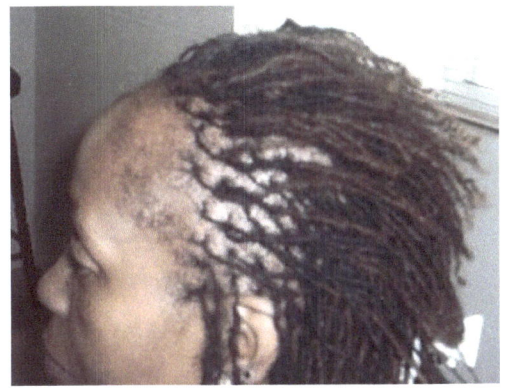 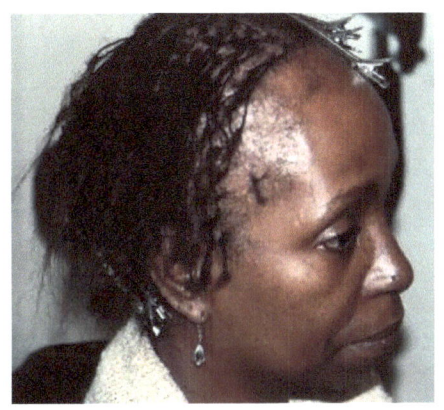

There was a colleague at work who had Sisterlocks^{tm} – very tiny Locs which I had never seen before. I inquired about her Locs and she told me how versatile they were.

I was growing my perm out and decided I needed a change. I found René online and made an appointment.

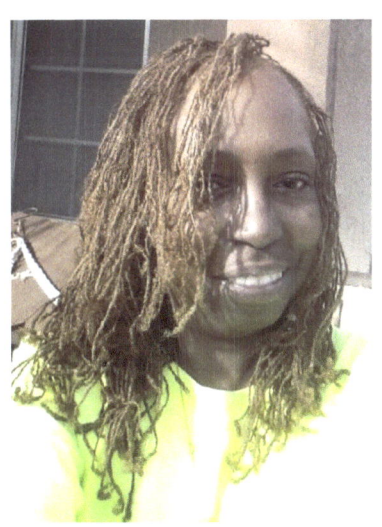

After our first session (my install), I wasn't sure and wondered, "what have I done!" My hair was very short and thin.

Over the months (and years), my hair has thickened and grown longer than I had initially imagined and is very versatile to style.

I love my hairstyle and wish I had done it sooner.

Dr. Gloria Bell, PhD

Author of 'Help for the Harvest'

My mother was my beautician until I went to college. I never worried about hair- how it looked, who would do it, when it would get done, until college life kicked in and 'do it yourself' became my mantra.

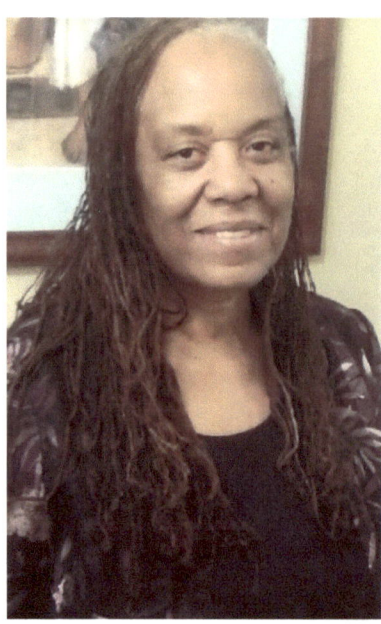

I tried pressing and curling which was more burning and frying. I tried perms from drug store box specials; more burning and frying was the result.

Finally, after graduating into real life and career, I turned to beauticians to 'fix my mess' and fix me an acceptable look.

While they did beautiful work, I was admittedly no good at styling. I just wanted a simple look that didn't require a lot of maintenance.

With a husband, three children and a teaching career, simple was all I could handle.

Over the years of over-processing and color-treating my hair, my glory was becoming my shame.

One day I met a friend that I hadn't seen in years. She told me that her beautiful Locs were called Sisterlocks^{tm}. It was love at first sight. She had curled them with rollers and they were beautiful and she looked gorgeous! I knew that this was what I've been looking for. I had to have Sisterlocks^{tm}.

She gave me the contact information and the rest is history. I have been totally excited and amazed at my Locs- 8 years and 30 inches later.

To me it's a miracle that my hair is actually continuously growing with near zero maintenance. And the styles are limitless.

Dr. Joscelin Thomas, PhD

My hair and I had a hate-hate relationship from a very young age.

My hair was thin and short and broke off a lot, especially in the top and front, where it shows the most.

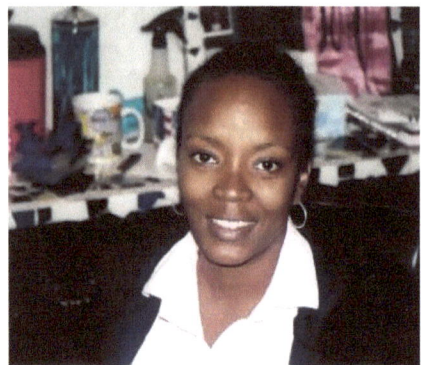

I was a sickly child, requiring a lot of medications and the relaxer and Jerri Curl made the condition of my hair very fragile, brittle and damaged. Like most girls my age, I wore braids a lot which also caused breaking.

Beautiful hair for me was impossible, even through my 20's. My hair was ugly and as a result so was I.

I was teased often because of my hair.

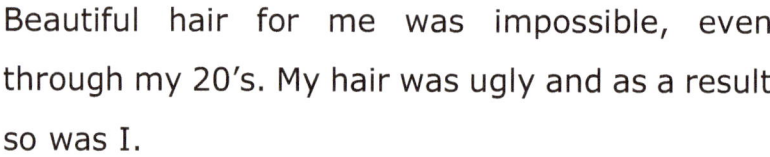

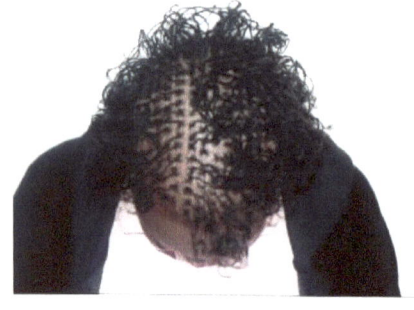

My natural hair journey started in 1999 when my aunt Monica was battling breast cancer. I cut off all my hair. I refused to allow anyone's view of beautiful hair define my beauty or that of my aunt anymore.

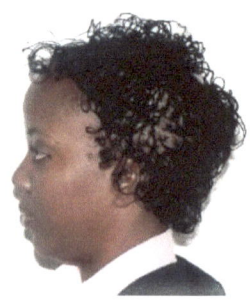

I wore a blonde fade for several years knowing that if and when I decided to let my hair grow back, I had to have a natural style.

I met so much resistance regarding my short hair; many opinions stating that my hair was my glory and that women displayed their beauty in their hair; REALLY? So, women are only beautiful if they have long hair? Processed hair?

Additions to their hair?

I wore my short hair a while longer making the statement that I was not hair struck.

It bothered me to hear people talk about good hair, bad hair, nappy hair etc.

Thinking back, I'm happy that I freed myself and my girls from the negativity connected to other people's view of my/our naturally beautiful hair.

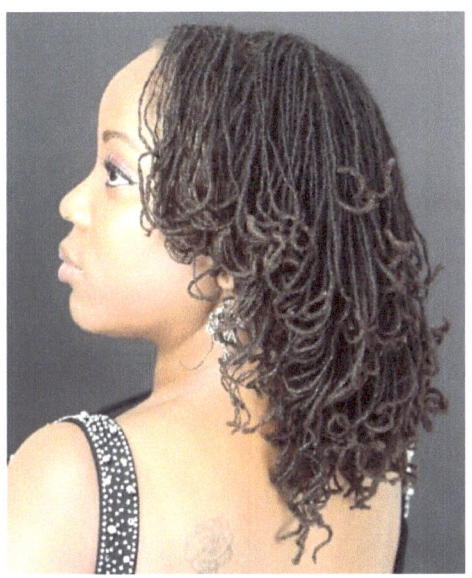 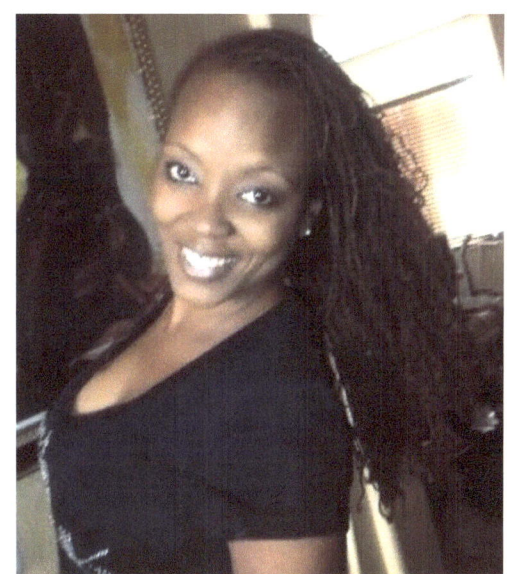

In 2005 I decided to grow my hair and begin the Sisterlocks™ journey and have never regretted my decision. October 26, 2005 I had my installation and have been free! René has been my consultant from the installation until now.

Jaelin Thomas

I like my natural hair in Sisterlocks^{tm} because it goes with me and it shows me for whom I am and I enjoy my Locs.

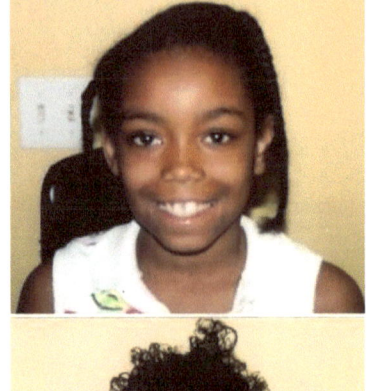

I like how I don't need to do them every day and they look pretty to me and on me in general.

My Locs make me look and feel sophisticated and therefore act like I am. People ask me why I have these and if I am ever going to cut them off. But I say, I have these because I wanted them and that I probably won't cut them.

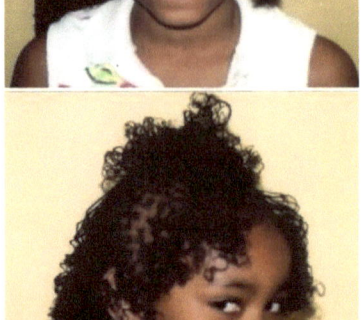

They also make me feel like my hair is getting longer and fuller. Also, since my hair is already long and luscious, it gives me more opportunities for new hair styles with this hair style and since Locs are kind of rare, it can be unique and very pretty.

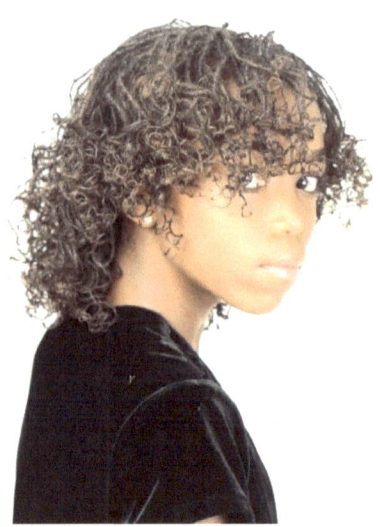 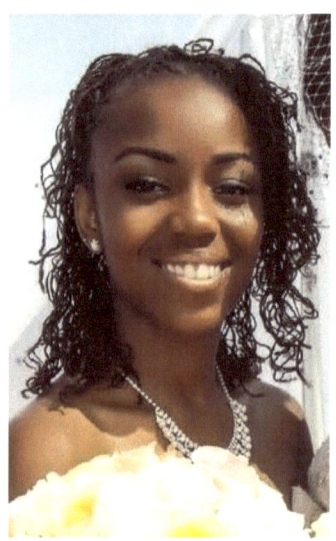 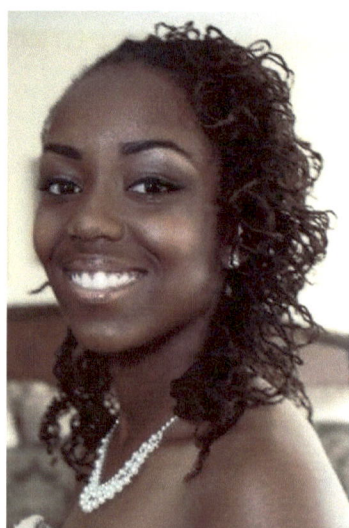

I love my natural hair and there is nothing anyone can say or do to change my mind.

Robin Allen

Prior to going 'Natural' I used to sit hours at the beauty shop on Saturdays and dreaded (no pun intended) every bit of it.

Once my hair was freshly done, I refused to exercise or do anything that would cause me to sweat. It took a great deal of time in the mornings to 'fix' my hair.

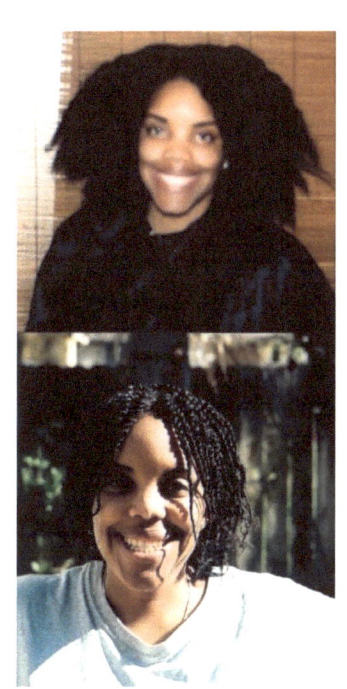

Management of my hair was too time consuming. I became tired of thinking about my hair and what to do about it. I wanted to go natural and wear Locs.

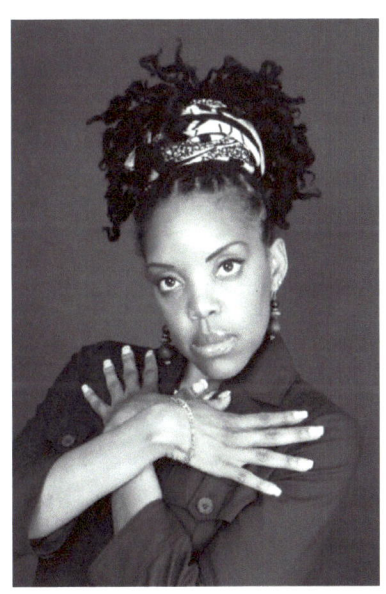

It took me a while to make the commitment initially.

I was afraid of cutting my hair should I decide I didn't want Locs anymore. I started with 2 strand twists (for about 6 months). I was comfortable with the look and decided to go all the way- 'let it dread'.

It's been 9 years without a bad hair day; 9 years of sweat and exercise; 9 years of hair freedom; 9 years of hair bliss!

I love my Locs. I feel authentic, natural, powerful and grateful for my Locs.

It make me giggle inside when people say, "wow, is all of that your hair?" Yes, it's all mine; all natural, never been cut or altered.

I do not own a comb or brush. I'm free- my Locs and I.

Paula Miller --Confessions of Picki-*Head* girl

I hated being called "picki-head" when I was growing up.

"Picki-head", a derogatory term used for having short thick kinky hair. Yep, I was called, *picki-head Paula*.

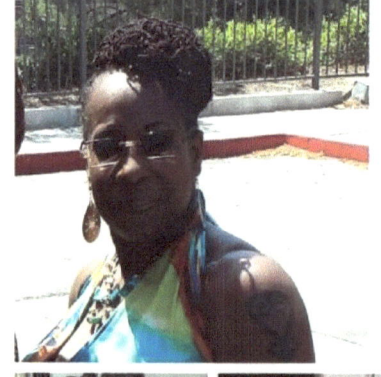

My hair was short and kinky and I hated it. My hair was so bad my mother sent me to get my hair pressed by miss Gloria and by the time I got home my hair was kinky again.

I hated my hair as a child. I spent lots of money trying to make my hair look right. Long hours at the hair salon; sometimes it became an all-day event. Even black hair dressers made it seem like our hair was raw leather.

Then, I discovered Sisterlocks[tm] and I said I am going to give this a try. My husband was quite encouraging and supportive of this decision.

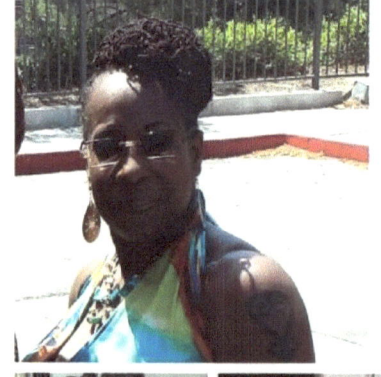
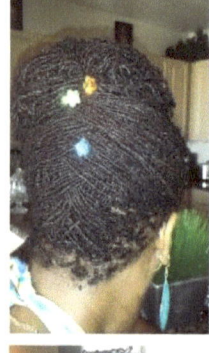

My picki-head turned into lovely Locs. Although the first day I came home, I looked at myself in the mirror and said, "OMG, what have I done?"

I looked a bit crazy but, I made it work. Then, my hair just started growing and my locks

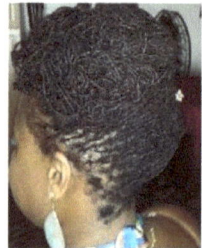
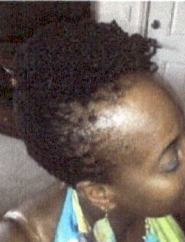
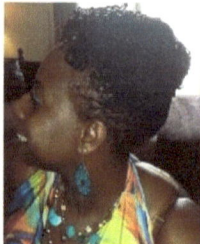

were beginning to have character and I was loving it.

50

I have kinky hair and I must say, I sure do love my hair now more than ever.

I no longer have to put a towel on my head pretending to have long hair like Wonder woman. I now have my own long hair that's kinky and thick and I love it!

Barbara L. Ray, Author, One of A Kind Vegetarian Cookbook/Divine Weight Loss Formula

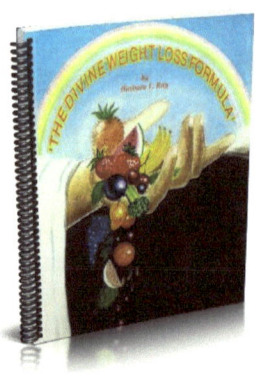

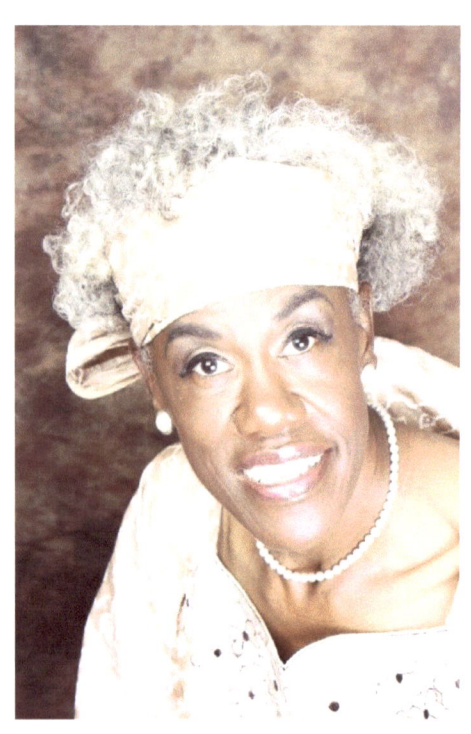

I decided to go *natural* because I started to embrace the natural beauty of my hair- a gift from God.

One of my hair horror stories was when I used to press my hair, and because it's gray, the heat from the pressing comb was turning my gray hair, brown—it was looking burnt! Now I do not press it. I wear it natural and kinky with discipline and care.

I found the right products and use them daily and faithfully. I am well pleased.

I feel great and free to be me. I don't have to compare my hair to anyone else's. I take care of it with love and appreciation and I feel Beautiful Hair® Products are the best products for me. It makes my gray hair soft, shiny and easy to manage as it grows and flows with life and strength!

Traci Daniels

My natural hair journey began when I finally became fed up after a 6 hour visit to the hair salon for a press and curl.

I had long given up perms due to the breakage it did to my hair, and I also had tried the streaks of color throughout my hair. It was beautiful in the beginning, but slowly continued to break off.

I had been seriously thinking about it and twist were becoming popular, so in 2007 I began going natural and doing my own twist.

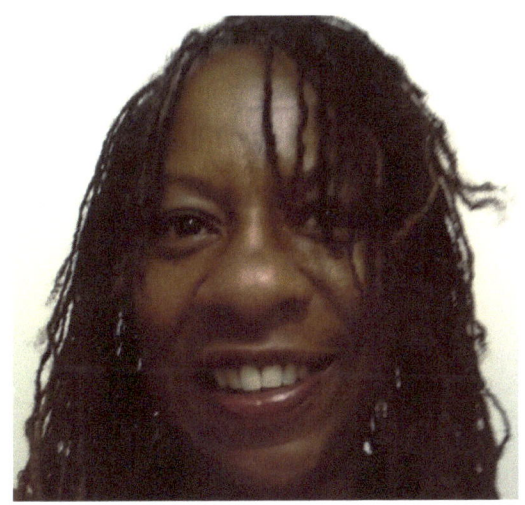

I was never a wig or weave lover because I like my scalp to breath!

I began growing out the ends of my perm/press with braids and cornrows and the twist. While all this was going on, menopause kicked in and more hair thinning.

I was already considering dreadlocks and then I began seeing women everywhere with these 'little dreads' and I knew it was for me.

In May 2010, I had a certified Sisterlocks^{tm} loctician put in my Locs, despite a friend stating, "men don't like that look." I simply love my Locs and don't care what anybody thinks.

I love the freedom, the beauty and the flexibility of my Locs and I continually get compliments.

My Locs have also inspired family members and friends to go natural and get Locs as well because they have also discovered that the hair God gave us *IS the Best hair*.

René began doing my Sisterlocks^{tm} in 2011 and she is truly a God-send. She not only nurtures your hair, she also nurtures your spirit.

LaShawnta Jackson

Approximately 3 years ago I was going on vacation and wanted 'worry free hair' so I had a weave sewn in. The kind of hair that is *soft and flowy* and

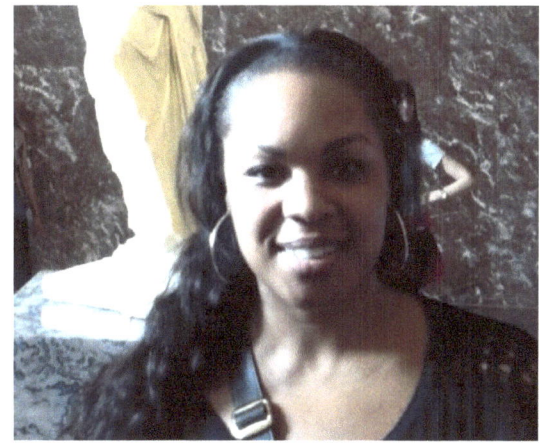

expensive enough that it would be downright embarrassing to say how much I actually spent.

After the weave was put in, I looked like I had a facelift and was so tight that I spent the first 3 days on medication for the headache (yeah, sad...I know).

A week into my vacation, my hair was still 'flowy', but there was a very tender spot in the center of my head. A week later, still sore; when I returned home I took the weave out along with a large scabby plug of my hair. This was the final straw. I was absolutely sick and tired of spending insane amounts of money for someone else's hair when I knew that my natural hair would be fine if I simply left it alone.

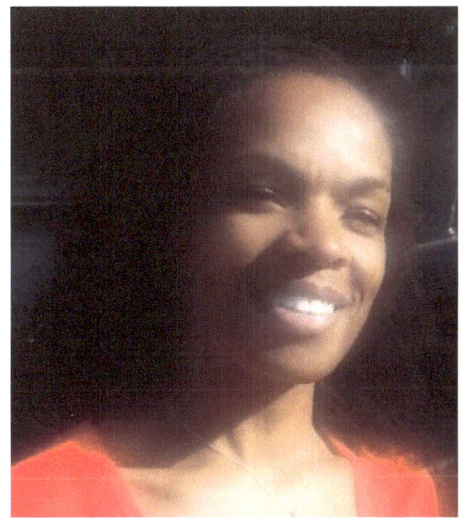

I made a pact with myself...I would wear my hair as natural as possible over the next 6 months (with as little heat as possible). I wanted to see if my natural hair could recover from all the heat, color, braiding, weaving, etc. over the past 30 years! And it did! I didn't die (although friends and family thought something was wrong with me because I was no longer wearing the weaves).

After another 6 months had passed and I became comfortable wearing two strand twists (that I did myself), I thought it was time to try Sisterlocks^{tm}. My hair has been growing like weeds ever since.

Sisterlocks^{tm} have been one of, if not the most liberating things I've done so far.

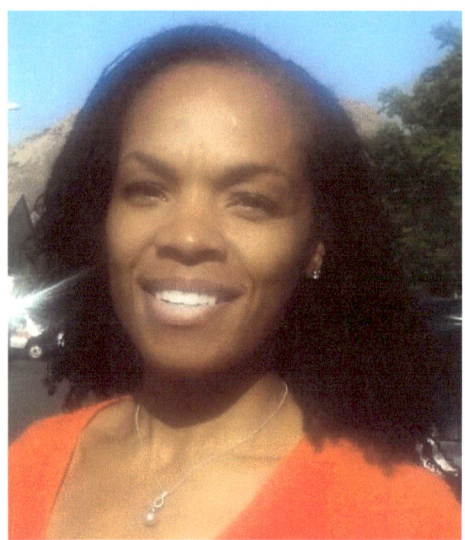

At this point, I don't ever see myself returning to the beauty supply, beauty salon rat race, awaiting some poor woman to chop off all her hair so that I can have it sewn on to my own!

Carla Thornton

I still remember being fourteen years old and getting a touch up on a perm. The hair dresser told me that although my hair had grown, my ends were very

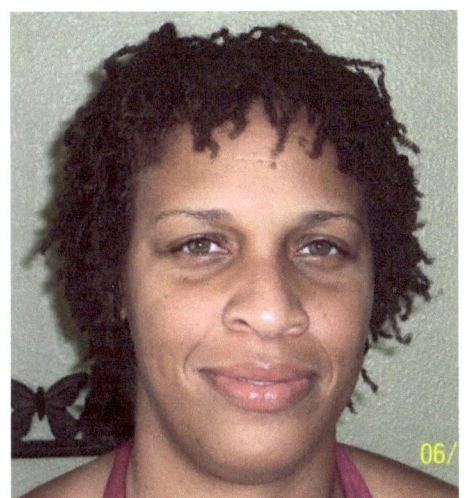

damaged and would have to be cut. She did my hair; when I went home to see how much she had cut, I sat in front of the mirror and cried. I felt so ugly.

For more than thirty years I went to hair dressers who told me my hair was "kinky, too fine, and hard to work with."

I struggled for years trying to make my hair do what it didn't want to do. And I was tired.

Although I loved braids and the variety of styles they offered, I got tired of having to take down the extensions and the endless hours sitting in the chair; I was looking for something- some way to wear my hair in a style that worked for the texture of my hair. Then one day my sister told me about Sisterlocks^{tm}.

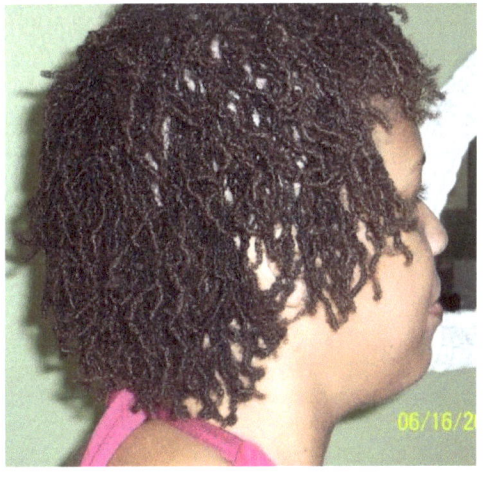

I watched videos and read chapters from books about black hair care. I started by wearing two strand twists. This was a huge leap for me. I had to embrace the more delicate look of my own hair…short, soft, kinky, but not silky or shiny. I knew that many people wouldn't like it, so I had to like it; I had to own it. And I did.

I wore my cork-screw-looking-twists for six months to get rid of the remainder of my last perm and got my Sisterlocks^{tm}. I was finally free!

I have been wearing the Locs for over five years, and I will continue to. For the first time when I sat in a stylist's chair- I was told, "your hair texture is perfect for Locs". No stylist had EVER said that to me. I felt happy, beautiful, comfortable...in short, I felt like myself.

I curl it, braid it, blow dry it, put bantu knots in it and I love all of it. I always feel good about my hair now. I feel that my hair is more than 'good'; it's

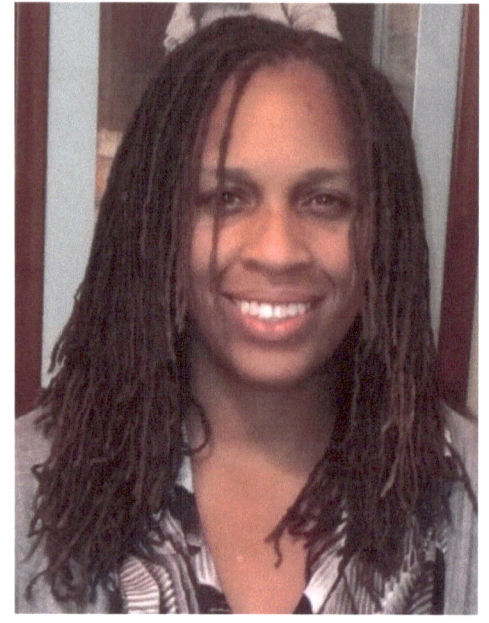

beautiful, because it's mine. It's healthy, strong, and natural.

It took me a long time to get to this place of being satisfied with my looks, and more importantly, my identity and self-concept as a black woman.

Wearing Sisterlocks^{tm} gives me so much confidence. No matter what I choose to wear, my look is distinctively me. And I am so fortunate to have René as my loctician whose products work so well to maintain the health of my hair. I continue to benefit from her skills, knowledge and products.

Healthy hair is beautiful hair.

Terri Thomas

In 2006, I went to a salon to get a hair-cut and relaxer. I ended up with over processed hair that was breaking off; the sides of my hair were approximately a half-inch short. Completely frustrated, and unsatisfied with the end result, I wore a bandana around my head to cover up my nearly shaved off sides for 2 months!

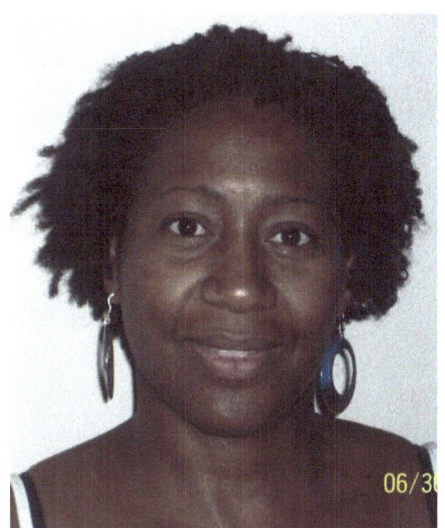

After numerous hair salon mishaps, I went on the African American cruise and saw several women who had Sisterlocks™, so I approached them to ask about how they like wearing them. They all stated that they 'loved' their hair. I came home and began meeting other women and did my research.

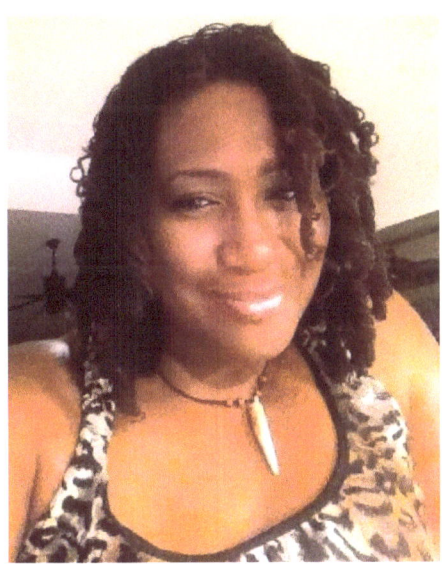
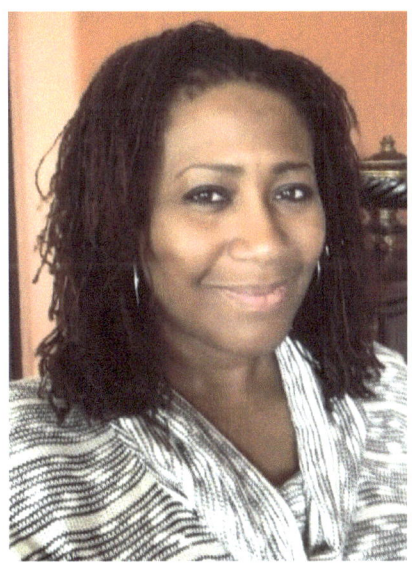

One year later I had decided to do it. I found René and have never left!

I am so in love with my hair and have found that I am even more comfortable with my own hair ~ I love my hair!

Karla Kimble

As a little girl, I dealt with what most little blacks girls deal with... kinky, coily, thick, coarse, nappy hair. You know the kind of hair that makes you run and

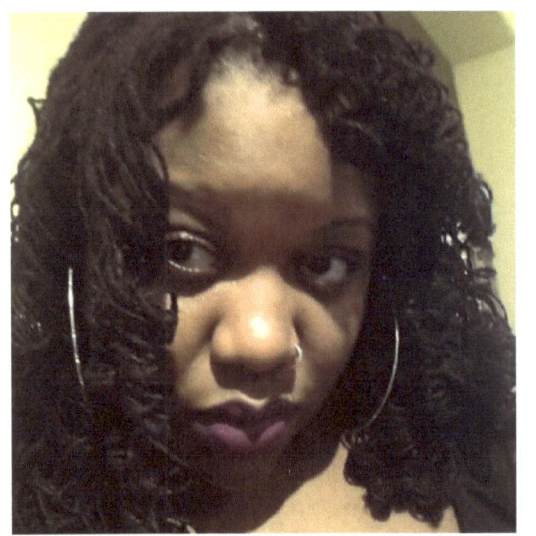

hide from a comb, because it was viewed as a torture device!

Most little black girls dream of having silky, flowing, long hair, the kind of hair that would make Rapunzel jealous, and I would be lying if I said that I was never one of them. I even remember being no more than 3 or 4 years old in dance school, and there were these 2 sisters, black girls, mixed with

Native American (I believe)... well they were sooo popular and everyone loved them, and would go on and on about their luxurious, beautiful, long and wavy hair, that flowed all the way down their backs! I was so consumed with wondering why I couldn't have hair like that!

So moving forward, I started with perms when I was around 9 years old I begged my mom for a *Just For Me* relaxer, and she finally gave in and allowed me to get a relaxer on my hair to make it *more manageable*.

After years and years of wearing chemical relaxers my scalp became extremely damaged and flaky, not to mention, hair breakage was horrible, especially in the crown and center vertex area of my head!

I teetered back and forth between braids and weaves, and just wearing my own natural hair in afros and puffs, etc.

I decided to finally go back to my natural hair in 2004, so I stopped putting chemicals in my hair, and cut off all of my permed ends...

I've always embraced my natural hair, and decided I wanted to get traditional Locs. I began an Internet search through Google, and found an array of beautiful styles... then I came across a picture of micro small Locs! They were beautiful!!! I found out they were called Sisterlocks™ and began a search on those. That's when I came across some gorgeous photos of Sisterlocks™ and it happened to be from Naturally Yours Boutique!

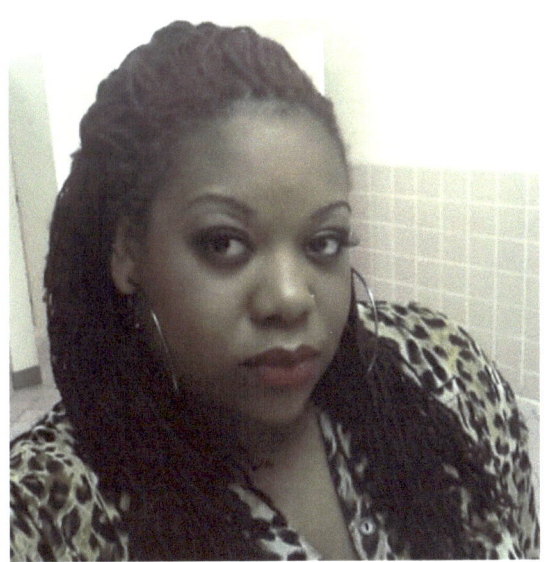 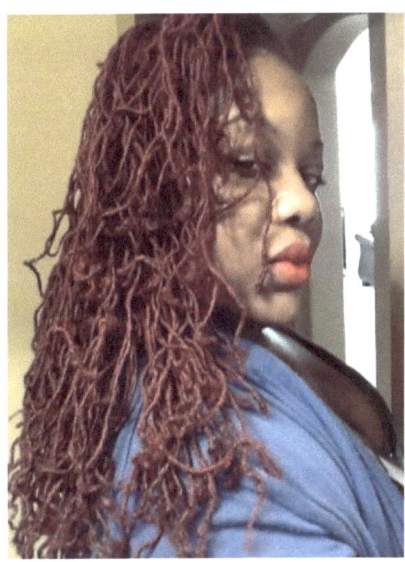

After doing some more research, I was all in! I was ready for my Sisterlocks™ journey to begin... and so I did on June 19, 2006; best decision (hair wise) that I ever made!

After 8 years, I still get amazing compliments on my hair! The ladies love them and the men can't keep their hands off them!

I feel so blessed to be living free and beautiful with my own natural head of hair, and I wouldn't have it any other way!

Quintin "*Kwame; Hitman_44*" Alexander

Professional Basketball player

I first got my dreads when I was 10 years old. But it wasn't necessarily my

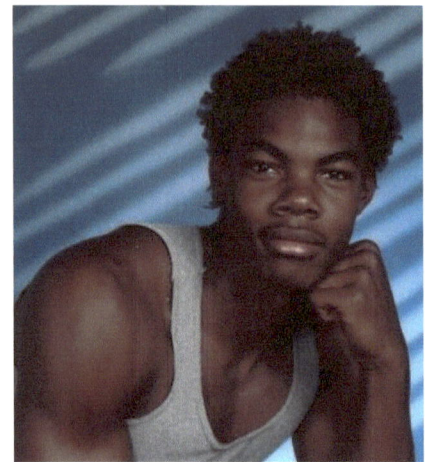

choice, my mom put them in my hair-- in all of our hair—me and my sisters. I wore them for 2 years and wanted to cut them off because I got tired of them. My mom had a fit! She tried to talk me out of cutting them, but my mind was made up. She reluctantly had my dad cut them off.

The summer before I went to the 11th grade I wanted them again, but this time it was my choice. I wanted Brotherlocks this time. They are much smaller than traditional dreadlocks.

I like my Locs because they're cool and give me a unique look.

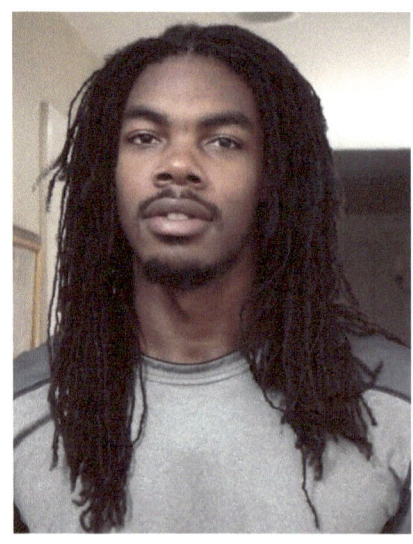
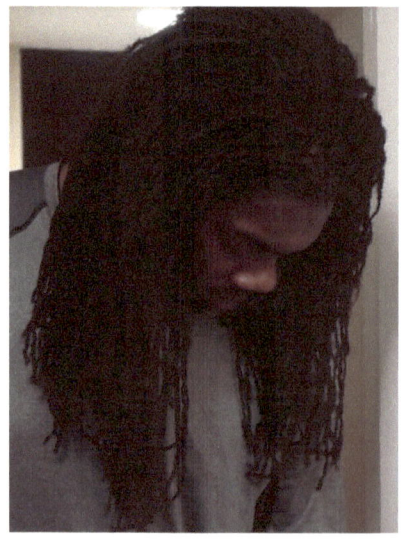

I'm a professional basketball player and my tiny Locs sets me apart from everybody else...plus I get a lot of attention from having my Locs.

Right now, I don't have any plans to ever cut my hair. I think my hair is cool and I'm glad to be in the 'loc' family.

Dr. Lakieta L. Emanuel

My Natural Hair Journey 13 year Update

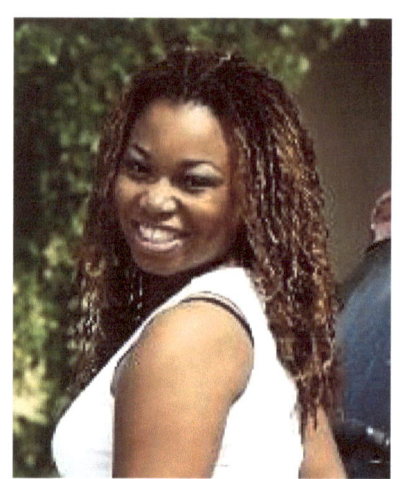

It seems just like yesterday when I decided to take the big step in becoming a part of the natural hair world. I had just gotten a relaxer so that my trip to Vegas to visit my parents would be met with acceptance from my mother. I looked in the mirror and put my hair in two pony tails and "snip", cut off the ends. When my husband arrived home from work, I asked him to use the shortest card and to shave my head as close as he could without leaving a bald shine.

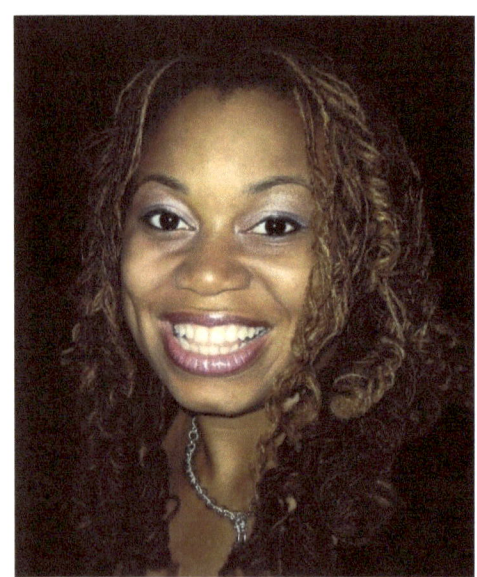

It's been 13 years since that monumental day. I look back at that brave 25 year old and think about how that one step toward wholeness has allowed me to take a million more in the direction of embracing all that God has naturally intended me to be.

My hair, over the last 13 years, has been trimmed, cut, dyed several times and has been in up-do's, twist-outs, curl formers, loc-loops, pipe cleaners. I have had a party with my hair and with myself. I am so glad I decided to love the hair that God gave me and once out of the proverbial "black woman's hair issues" box, I will never go back. I love that I can work out, swim, and take a stroll in the rain without care or panic over hair.

Something even greater has come most unexpectedly from that decision I made to love my hair. All of my close friends have decided to do the same. My sister is now natural, and all of my mentee's. To me this is the best part. The lesson is that when you love yourself, you indirectly give others the permission to do the same. I love my hair, now and forever!!

René Michelle Floyd

CEO Founder and Owner of Naturally Yours Boutique, Inc.

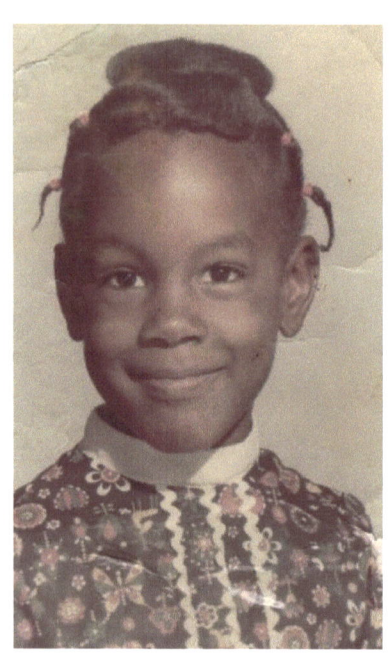

Picture day was exciting for me because I got to wear my famous "bangs"—I got to wear my hair "pressed". My mother would screw what little hair I had tightly into those infamous rubber bands and neatly braid my inch and a half hair, so that I would look nice for my glamour shot school pictures.

One day, I was playing with my friend (I was about 8 years old) and her mother made a comment about my hair that affected my self-esteem and perception of my hair for years to come..."look at René's little short hair"...to this day I don't remember what she was talking about and why she would say something like that, all I know is that I stormed out her house wailing and crying with my feelings hurt as if someone had slapped me in the face! I went crying to my mother...I could hardly contain myself enough to talk. I didn't understand why I was so affected like that at the time, but I was.

For years after that I went on a quest to "get some long hair". I wore ponytail attachments, wigs, extension braids, loc extensions, you name it, and I did it! I tried everything to look like everybody else only to suffer the pain of a sore scalp and damaged hair. I kept having to cut my hair off and start over again with braids to grow out my hair, just to repeat that same old vicious cycle.

One day, I had a revelation...God revealed to me that Locs was my style—it agreed with my hair. I would have freedom and my hair would grow stronger and longer than ever. So I braided my hair and left the braids in for months—my hair started to dread and this was the start of my "new" hairstyle.

My hair was doing fine and growing nicely for 5 years...until, one day I had

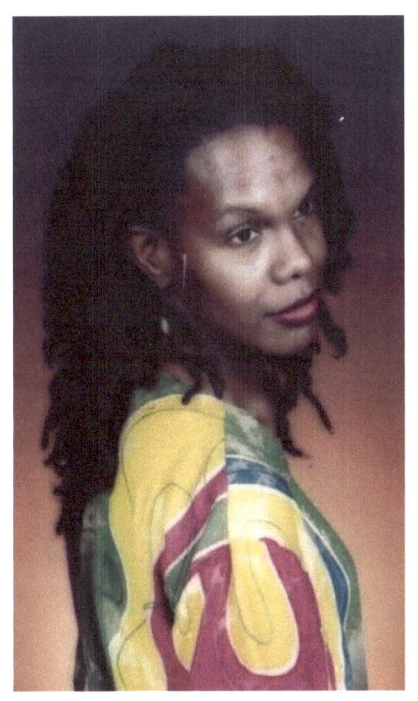

this idea that I wanted volume and fullness to my perceived, thin hair—so I wrapped human hair around each dreadlock and created-- 'loc extensions'—my hair was beautiful and full—

BUT as my hair grew out, the weight of the added hair started pulling my hair and breaking off...about this time I saw someone with Sisterlocks ᵗᵐ and loved them. I scheduled a consultation. I took out one of the extensions in order to put test Locs in. I really liked how the Sisterlocks ᵗᵐ looked and felt—I wanted them...so, I went home to take the rest of the extensions out so that I could wash and

condition my hair in preparation for my Sisterlocks ᵗᵐ (so I thought). Those extensions weren't budging! Those things were impossible to take out—so guess what I did? Yes, I cut out all those Locs and again, there I was at square one with one and a half inches of hair!

Before I got my Sisterlocks ᵗᵐ installed, I decided I wanted more length to my hair, so I braided my hair to grow it out (once again) and my hair did grow.

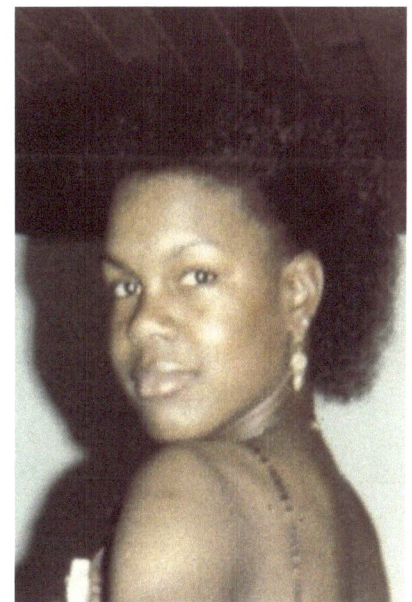

One day, as my hair was in its' "recovery" state, I got this idea (crazy idea) that I wanted a braid weave, so I put individual small human hair braids in my "recovering fragile" hair. I went to the "beauty shop" and got a cute cut.

Off and running I went—about three weeks into my "new" style, my hair began to break again because of all the finger combing, pulling and dryness of my hair while running my fingers through it. My hair was very dry and breaking out in patches. Back to square one again! When was I going to ever learn?

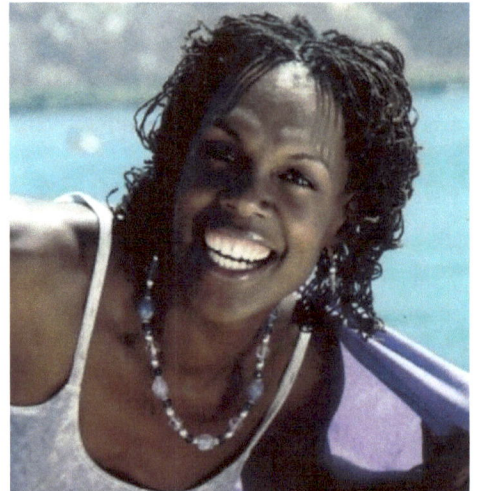

Finally, I gave up and just started tying my hair up with pretty African clothe (while my hair grew back).

I went to the Sisterlocks^{tm} training class to become a Sisterlocks^{tm} consultant; all the while I was going to class, I was so embarrassed about my hair—I kept it tied up—no one saw my hair—my class mates and the instructor encouraged me to go ahead and get Sisterlocks^{tm}. "Sisterlocks^{tm} will help your hair grow and heal faster," they said, but I was adamant on having 'length' before I put my Sisterlocks^{tm} in—so I didn't listen. Finally a couple months went by and I got tired of tying my hair up--besides, it didn't seem to be growing as fast as I knew it could had I gotten the Sisterlocks^{tm} earlier. I broke down and called Michelle and asked her to rescue me— she happened to have an appointment open and took me the next day...my saving grace! My hair was so broken and damaged. I don't know how Michelle was even able to catch some of my hair to lock it (she has gifted hands).

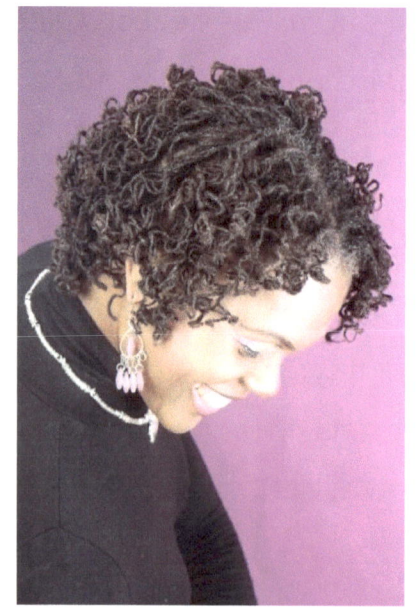

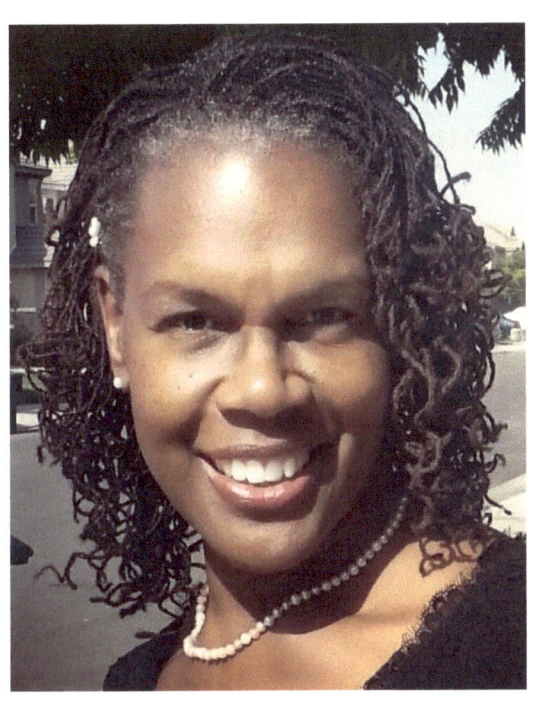

Getting Sisterlocks™ was the best decision I could have made for my hair...today my hair is healthier than ever and is growing past the bottom of my neck—and the best part is that it's all mine! NO extensions, NO attachments—all me and I'm lovin' it! I can't wait till my hair is 'flowing' down the middle of my back!

RESOURCES & INFORMATION

Beautiful Hair Products

Exclusively from Naturally Yours Boutique, Inc.

http://www.Store.NaturallyYoursBoutique.com

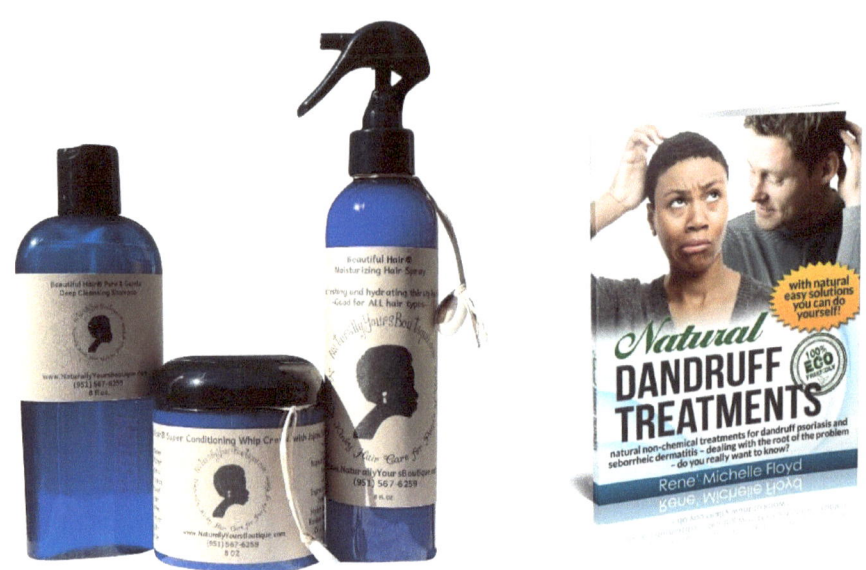

- Beautiful Hair Super Conditioning Whip Crème w/Jojoba Oil & Lanolin— 8 oz. jar
- Moisturizing Hair Spray—8 oz.
- Pure & Gentle Deep Cleansing Shampoo
- Natural Dandruff Treatments book
- And More!

**For more information on how to treat dandruff naturally and how to purchase *Natural Green Products* contact René Michelle Floyd directly at: (951) 567-6259 or directly via email: Rene@NaturallyYoursBoutique.com

One of a Kind Vegetarian Cookbook

AND

The Divine Weight Loss Formula

By Barbara L. Ray

Two books in one!

http://www.TheDivineWeightLossFormula.com

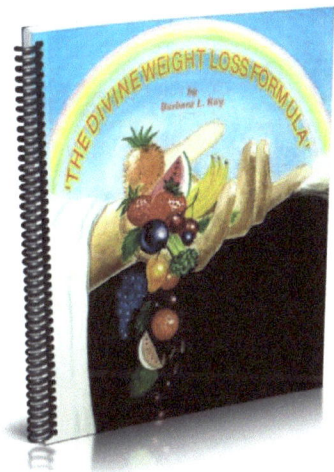

One of A Kind Vegetarian Cookbook AND The Divine Weight Loss Formula by Barbara L. Ray (Health Consultant and Vegan) is a Combined edition! Two books in one! Filled with delicious vegetarian recipes and fresh juice recipes that is simple and easy to make. A great book for those desiring to transition into a healthier way of cooking…you will find a food plan and menu included…of course, a healthy head of hair is directly linked to the diet you eat and the liquid you drink…very informative and simple. OKVC and TDWLF book is *a must!*

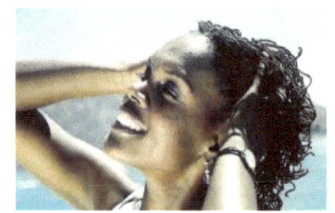

EMBRACING YOUR BEAUTY...from the INSIDE OUT---COMPACT DISC (CD) or MP3 Download

We as women have such a wonderful 'natural' quality about us, which sometimes get 'lost' in the 'worlds' we create for ourselves.

Embracing Your Beauty...from the Inside Out is one of the most uplifting, affirming, inspirational, and motivational set of messages you've probably heard in quite some time. Its' purpose is to usher you into self-acceptance, love and peace.

You are going to fall in love with yourself all over again...and for some-- for the first time. Truly in order to love someone else you must love yourself first—

"Love your neighbor as you love yourself"—how can we, if we don't love ourselves? Well, that is about to change—

A few testimonials--

- "Very empowering...uplifting...going to raise the consciousness of many women—and men also".

---Shirley R. --- Ontario, California

- "The esteem and spirit of all human beings is a crucial part of growing and developing as a person. As I was having my hair (Brother Locks) retightened and "threaded" from the root of my scalp at Naturally Yours Boutique, I heard the recorded words of (René Michelle Floyd AKA- Olufemi Alexander) fall upon my ears. The words were ones of encouragement and self-identity: To love one's self despite the backbiting of the external world and for Wo-man (woman and man/female and male energy) to find the thread of unity that maintains the balance of life on earth. Readily, all six tracks of spoken 'affirmations' of self-respect and beauty (inside and out), reach out immediately to the female person listening, and all reiterations of dignity/self-worth she has and should continue to share on planet earth.

In addition, the female part of all who listen to René's words can strengthen the masculine sensibilities of the man who hears the words of 'respect', 'dignity', 'care', 'joy', 'life', and 'love', recited by natural hair and natural care loctician, René Michelle Floyd.

In closing, respectful sounds that sway forth through the air that accompany any unifying and self-respecting words of woman/man and their sense of black or African ness, as put forth sensitively by René, is a blessing." --Rashad S. ---Riverside, California

- "Listening to, "Embracing Your Beauty...from the Inside Out", was a spirit lifter for me. Now I see the beauty in me from the inside out. Thank you, my daughter René Michelle Floyd for this wonderful CD."

---Barbara L. Ray----Moreno Valley, California

- "Very uplifting...reminded me of who I am—I am somebody; I have purpose...encouraging to my mind, body and soul...feel the peace of the speaker. Serenity, love, life, comfort."

----Lovie S. ----Riverside, California

Grab your copy TODAY and begin your NEW-found love affair with yourself, the way God intended. www.CDBaby.com/OlufemiAmusic

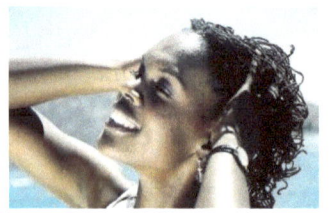

"Embracing Your Beauty...from the Inside Out"

www.CDBaby.com/OlufemiAmusic

The compact disk version $12.97 (plus S/H) or **_MP3 instant download!_** Only $6 Bucks!!!

Download to your computer, iPod or MP3 player and begin listening and enjoying within minutes!!!

Social Connections

Beautiful Hair Products & Accessories Store

http://www.Store.NaturallyYoursBoutique.com

- **Tweet Us**: http://twitter.com/nybinc

- **Facebook Us:** http://facebook.com/ReneMichelleFloyd

- **Facebook Us:** http://facebook.com/BeautifulHairProducts

- **Watch Us**: http://youtube.com/ReneMFloyd

- **Link to Us**: http://LinkedIn.com/in/ReneMichelleFloyd

G+ (Google Plus): https://plus.google.com/+ReneMichelleFloydnyb

My other books can be found on Amazon at:

http://www.amazon.com/Rene-Michelle-Floyd/e/B006EU0K4Q

www.ingramcontent.com/pod-product-compliance
Lightning Source LLC
Chambersburg PA
CBHW041500280526
45792CB00004B/1073